To my dear sister
Arlene Elizabeth Becker
Christmas 1999

At Last—Down-Home Food Diabetics Can Enjoy, Too!

By Kathy Redlinger, Registered Dietitian and Certified Diabetes Educator

AS SOMEONE who's spent her life helping people make good nutritional choices and working with those on special diets, I'm excited by the publication of this long-needed book.

For years, those with diabetes—and others who are limiting their intake of calories, fat, cholesterol and sodium—have faced a difficult choice several times a day. They could carefully follow the too-often bland-tasting diet their doctor placed them on...or they could ignore their doctor's advice and continue to eat the hearty stick-to-your-ribs meals they'd long enjoyed.

That was the unhappy choice, that is, *until now*. This book, the *Down-Home Diabetic Cookbook*, breaks new ground by making it possible to enjoy deliciously filling farm-style meals (potato dumpling soup, pork stew, hamburger casserole, etc.) and treats (cookies, cakes, ice cream and—yes—even pies) while still following a diabetic diet. You'll feel like you're "splurging" on your diet...but you won't be!

That's because the *Down-Home Diabetic Cookbook* is packed with 300 of the "real food for real people" type of recipes found in every issue of North America's most popular cooking magazine, *Taste of Home*. The only difference is that *every one* of the recipes in this book also meets the needs of those on special diets.

In many cases, they are proven "lighter" favorites of a particular cook's family. In others, home economists have adjusted the ingredients of treasured old-fashioned recipes to meet the needs of those on special diets. Whatever the case, each recipe has been thoroughly tested in the Reiman Publications Test Kitchen *and* personally reviewed by me to ensure it meets all the qualifications required of a special-diet recipe.

Here are a few other things to keep in mind about this unique cookbook:

● Every recipe includes nutritional analysis *and* diabetic exchanges. Exchanges are based on the standards set by the American Diabetes Association and the American Dietetic Association.

● Occasionally, you'll find a "special treat"—take the Sugar-Free Apple Pie on page 304, for example. That recipe fits the bill for low-sugar cooking. However, keep in mind that because of the pastry crust, the fat grams will be higher than in other restricted diet recipes. So, while not intended for everyday use, such recipes are perfect for special occasions!

● Those especially concerned with sodium intake will note that recipes using canned foods are higher in sodium than those using all fresh ingredients. So be sure to select recipes that fit your individual restrictions. At the same time, though, keep an eye out while grocery shopping for new products that have reduced sodium or no salt added. Helpful products like that regularly become available, expanding the range of recipes those with diet restrictions can use. As they do, feel free to substitute them for similar higher-sodium ingredients where appropriate.

● Sugar *is* used in some recipes in this book. Why? Experts now agree that sugar may be used *in limited amounts* by *most* people with diabetes. Whenever sugar is used in a recipe in this cookbook, it is included in the carbohydrate value used to calculate the diabetic exchange.

● Finally—and most importantly—if you have questions about using sugar, or any other questions about your diet, special restrictions and how the recipes in this book fit into your individual program, contact your dietitian or doctor.

CONTENTS

Editor: Julie Schnittka
Food Editor: Mary Beth Jung
Assistant Food Editor: Coleen Martin
Dietitian: Kathy Redlinger, R.D.
Art Director: Ellen Lloyd
Associate Editors: Kristine Krueger, Henry de Fiebre
Test Kitchen Home Economists: Rochelle Schmidt, Karla Spies
Test Kitchen Assistants: Judith Scholovich, Sherry Smalley
Photography: Scott Anderson, Mike Huibregtse
Prop Stylist: Anne Schimmel
Illustrations: Jim Sibilski

©1995, Reiman Publications, L.P.
5400 S. 60th Street, Greendale WI 53129
International Standard Book Number 0-89821-153-0
Library of Congress Number: 95-71713
All rights reserved. Printed in U.S.A.

Snacks & Beverages

After tasting these delicious dips, spreads and beverages, you'll agree that anytime snacking has never been better.

Pineapple Smoothie

Margery Bryan, Royal City, Washington

*I've tried several diabetic beverage recipes through the years.
I found this pineapple drink recipe 20 years ago and
it's still one of the best I've ever had.*

1 can (20 ounces) pineapple chunks
   in natural juices
1 cup buttermilk
2 teaspoons vanilla extract
2 teaspoons liquid artificial
   sweetener
Mint leaves, optional

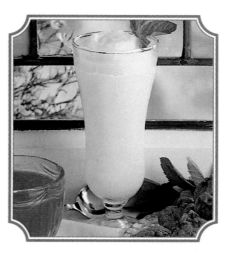

Drain pineapple, reserving 1/2 cup juice.
Freeze pineapple chunks. Place juice, buttermilk, vanilla, sweetener and frozen
pineapple into a blender container. Blend
until smooth. Pour into glasses and garnish with mint if desired. Serve immediately. **Yield:** 5 servings.

Exchanges: 1/2 Skim Milk, 1/2 Fruit
Nutritional Information

Serving Size: 1/5 recipe
Calories: 74
Sodium: 52 mg
Cholesterol: 2 mg

Carbohydrate: 16 gm
Protein: 2 gm
Fat: 1 gm

Curried Chicken Cheese Ball

Pauline Rhine, Bunker Hill, Indiana

I cater for parties, so I'm always searching for new menu ideas that fit into everyone's diet. I discovered a similar cheese ball recipe in a magazine, then adjusted the ingredients to suit my tastes.

1 package (8 ounces) **light cream cheese, softened**
2 tablespoons orange marmalade
1-1/2 teaspoons curry powder
1/4 teaspoon white pepper
2 cups finely chopped cooked chicken
2 tablespoons minced green onions
2 tablespoons minced celery
3/4 cup chopped fresh parsley

In a mixing bowl, beat cream cheese, marmalade, curry powder and pepper until smooth. Stir in chicken, onions and celery. Shape into a large ball. Roll in parsley. Cover and chill. Serve with crackers. **Yield:** 10 servings (2 cups).

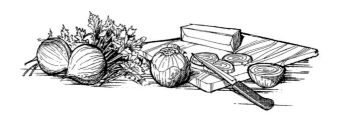

Exchanges: 1/2 Meat, 1/2 Fat, 1/2 Fruit
Nutritional Information

Serving Size: 3 tablespoons
Calories: 89
Sodium: 135 mg
Cholesterol: 30 mg

Carbohydrate: 5 gm
Protein: 7 gm
Fat: 5 gm

White Bean Dip

Linn Landry, Honeydew, California

Most store-bought bean dips are loaded with preservatives, not to mention fat. So this homemade low-fat version was a welcome addition to my recipe file.

1 can (15 to 16 ounces) cannellini beans *or* great northern beans, rinsed and drained
1 tablespoon lemon juice
2 tablespoons plain fat-free yogurt
2 tablespoons chopped fresh parsley
1/2 teaspoon freshly ground black pepper
1/4 teaspoon hot pepper sauce
2 to 3 garlic cloves

In a food processor or blender, combine all ingredients. Cover and process until smooth. Chill. Serve with toasted pita bread, corn chips or fresh vegetables. **Yield:** 1-1/4 cups.

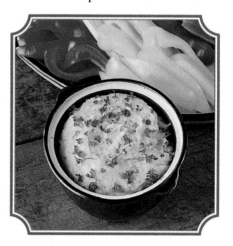

Exchanges: 1/2 Starch

Nutritional Information

Serving Size: 1 tablespoon
Calories: 29
Sodium: 78 mg
Cholesterol: trace

Carbohydrate: 6 gm
Protein: 2 gm
Fat: trace

Sugar-Free Cocoa Mix

Marion Kowalski, Wauwatosa, Wisconsin

During the winter, I keep plenty of this mix on hand. That way, I can whip up steaming mugs of hot cocoa as soon as the kids come in from playing outside.

2 cups nonfat dry milk powder
1/2 cup low-fat powdered nondairy creamer
1/2 cup baking cocoa
10 packets artificial sweetener (equivalent to 3 tablespoons sugar)
3/4 teaspoon ground cinnamon

Combine all of the ingredients. Store in an airtight container. For each serving, add 1/3 cup mix to 3/4 cup boiling water; stir to dissolve. **Yield:** 2-2/3 cups mix (8 servings).

STRAIGHT FROM THE HEART. Think that you can't give diabetic friends a holiday gift from your kitchen? Well, you can! Just make a batch of this Sugar-Free Cocoa Mix, put it in a festive jar and wrap it with the directions attached. They'll thank you for remembering them.

Exchanges: 1 Milk
Nutritional Information

Serving Size: 1 cup
Calories: 104
Sodium: 93 mg
Cholesterol: 3 mg

Carbohydrate: 17 gm
Protein: 8 gm
Fat: 2 gm

Shrimp Spread

Norene Wright, Manilla, Indiana

This colorful and tasty appetizer is always a crowd-pleaser whenever I take it to potlucks and picnics. With such rich flavor, people will never know you've used lighter ingredients.

1 package (8 ounces) light cream cheese, softened
1/2 cup light sour cream
1/4 cup light mayonnaise
1 cup seafood cocktail sauce
2 cups (8 ounces) shredded light mozzarella cheese
2 cans (4-1/4 ounces *each*) shrimp, rinsed and drained
3 green onions, sliced
3/4 cup finely chopped tomato

In a small mixing bowl, beat the cream cheese, sour cream and mayonnaise until smooth. Spread on a 12-in. round serving platter. Cover with seafood sauce. Sprinkle with cheese, shrimp, onions and tomato. Cover and chill. Serve with crackers. **Yield:** 10 servings.

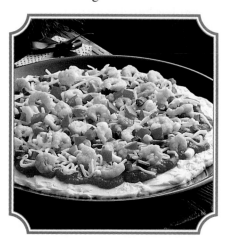

Exchanges: 1 Fat

Nutritional Information

Serving Size: 2 tablespoons
Calories: 38
Sodium: 112 mg
Cholesterol: 12 mg

Carbohydrate: 2 gm
Protein: 2 gm
Fat: 2 gm

Sugar-Free Holiday Nog

Nancy Schickling, Bedford, Virginia

Coming up with holiday beverages for someone who's diabetic can be a real challenge. This nog is so refreshing you'll be tempted to make it throughout the year!

1 package (.9 ounce) sugar-free instant vanilla pudding mix
7 cups skim milk, *divided*
1 to 2 teaspoons vanilla extract
  ***or* rum flavoring**
2 to 4 packets artificial sweetener
1 cup evaporated skim milk

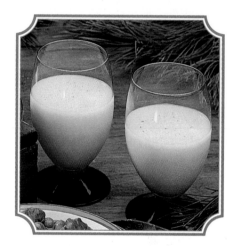

Combine pudding mix, 2 cups of milk, vanilla and sweetener in a bowl; mix according to pudding directions. Pour into a 1/2-gal. container with a tight-fitting lid. Add 3 cups milk; shake well. Add evaporated milk and shake. Add remaining milk; shake well. Chill. **Yield:** 8 servings.

Exchanges: 1 Skim Milk, 1/4 Starch

Nutritional Information

Serving Size: 1 cup
Calories: 107
Sodium: 187 mg
Cholesterol: 1 mg

Carbohydrate: 15 gm
Protein: 10 gm
Fat: 1 gm

Fruit Punch

Ruth Tacoma, Falmouth, Michigan

We had a diabetic child in our church youth group a few years ago and I tried to fix snacks that would be within his restrictions but enjoyable for the other kids as well. This punch really fills the bill.

1 package (.35 ounce) sugar-free tropical punch-flavored soft drink mix
4-3/4 cups water
1 can (12 ounces) unsweetened frozen orange juice concentrate, thawed
4 quarts diet white soda

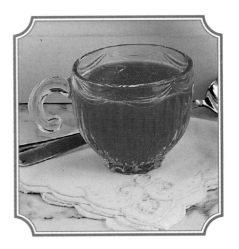

In a large pitcher, combine soft drink mix and water; mix well. Add orange juice concentrate; mix well. When ready to serve, pour into punch bowl and add the white soda. **Yield:** 20 servings (5 quarts).

COOL IDEA. When serving fruit juices or punch, try making ice cubes from the drinks. This will keep the beverages from becoming watered down.

Exchanges: 1/2 Fruit

Nutritional Information

Serving Size: 1 cup
Calories: 38
Sodium: 3 mg
Cholesterol: 0

Carbohydrate: 9 gm
Protein: trace
Fat: trace

Crunchy Chicken Balls

Jamie Cox, Chatham, Virginia

Now that I'm retired from teaching, I have plenty of time to cook and entertain. These individual chicken balls are always on the menu...much to the pleasure of my guests.

  1 cup finely chopped cooked chicken
1/4 cup minced green onions
1/2 cup finely shredded low-fat sharp
    cheddar cheese
1/8 teaspoon pepper
  2 tablespoons light mayonnaise
3/4 cup chopped fresh parsley

In a bowl, combine the first five ingredients; mix well. Shape into 3/4-in. balls. Roll in parsley. Cover and chill. **Yield:** 8 servings (2 dozen).

AVOID OVERCOOKING. Chicken cooked in the microwave will be moist and juicy if it is covered and cooked for the proper amount of time. Estimate 7 minutes per pound for a whole chicken and 5 minutes per pound if cut up.

Exchanges: 1 Lean Meat
Nutritional Information

Serving Size: 3 chicken balls
Calories: 49
Sodium: 79 mg
Cholesterol: 16 mg

Carbohydrate: 2 gm
Protein: 5 gm
Fat: 3 gm

Zucchini/Herb Pate

Melissa Sullivan, Iuka, Kansas

A friend gave me the recipe for this pate after she'd served it at a formal wedding reception. But I make it most often to spread on crackers at picnics, potlucks and other casual get-togethers.

4 medium zucchini (about 1 pound)
2 teaspoons tarragon vinegar
2 teaspoons sugar
2 teaspoons salt, *divided*
1/2 cup packed fresh parsley sprigs
1/2 cup snipped fresh chives *or*
1/4 cup dried chives
1 package (8 ounces) light cream cheese, softened
1/2 teaspoon pepper

Line a mixing bowl with a double thickness of cheesecloth. Coarsely shred zucchini into prepared bowl. Sprinkle with vinegar, sugar and 1 teaspoon salt. Toss gently; cover with a towel and set aside for 1 hour. Meanwhile, in a food processor with the chopping blade, mince parsley and chives. Gather ends of cheesecloth, squeezing out as much liquid as possible. Add drained zucchini to food processor and process until pureed. Add cream cheese, pepper and remaining salt; process until smooth. Press pate into a small bowl. Cover and refrigerate overnight. Serve with crackers. **Yield:** 1-1/2 cups.

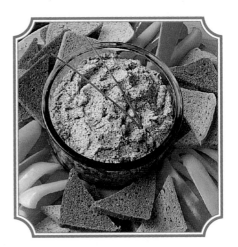

Exchanges: 1/2 Vegetable, 1/2 Fat

Nutritional Information

Serving Size: 1 tablespoon
Calories: 29
Sodium: 280 mg
Cholesterol: 5 mg

Carbohydrate: 3 gm
Protein: 2 gm
Fat: 2 gm

Cappuccino Shake

Paula Pelis, Rocky Point, New York

I created this quick and easy shake for my mom, who's been diabetic for 30 years. She was tickled pink! And now when I want to "indulge", I'll reach for this wonderful recipe.

1 cup skim milk
1-1/2 teaspoons instant coffee crystals
2 packets artificial sweetener (equivalent to 4 teaspoons sugar)
2 drops brandy extract *or* rum extract
Dash ground cinnamon

In a blender, combine milk, coffee crystals, sweetener and extract. Blend until coffee is dissolved. Serve with a dash of cinnamon. For a hot drink, pour into a mug and heat in a microwave. **Yield:** 1 serving.

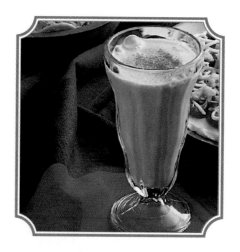

SPICE IT UP! If you serve this Cappuccino Shake hot, offer cinnamon sticks as stirrers. Everyone will love the added flavor.

Exchanges: 1 Milk
Nutritional Information

Serving Size: 1 cup
Calories: 100
Sodium: 128 mg
Cholesterol: 4 mg

Carbohydrate: 15 gm
Protein: 9 gm
Fat: trace

'Broccomole' Dip

Sue Gronholz, Columbus, Wisconsin

For a snack that's very much like guacamole—but without the avocados, which are high in fat—try this dip. I grow and freeze broccoli, so this recipe is convenient to make.

2 cups chopped fresh broccoli, cooked and chilled
1/4 cup light sour cream
1 to 2 tablespoons minced onion
1 tablespoon fat-free mayonnaise
2 to 3 tablespoons lemon juice
1/4 to 1/2 teaspoon chili powder

In a food processor or blender, combine all ingredients and blend until smooth. Refrigerate for several hours. Serve with fresh vegetables or baked tortilla chips. **Yield:** 6 servings.

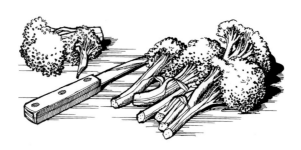

Exchanges: 1 Vegetable

Nutritional Information

Serving Size: 3 tablespoons
Calories: 27
Sodium: 33 mg
Cholesterol: 5 mg

Carbohydrate: 3 gm
Protein: 2 gm
Fat: 2 gm

Tomato Vegetable Juice

Sue Wille, Alexandria, Minnesota

I've used this delicious recipe for many years, and it's always been a favorite. The tangy juice is refreshing on its own and also works great in any recipe calling for tomato juice. Because of all the vegetables, it's full of vitamins.

10 pounds tomatoes, peeled and chopped (about 8 quarts)
3 garlic cloves, minced
2 large onions, chopped
2 carrots, cut into 1/2-inch slices
2 cups chopped celery
1/2 cup chopped green pepper
1/4 cup sugar
1 teaspoon Worcestershire sauce
1/2 teaspoon pepper
Lemon juice

Combine tomatoes, garlic, onions, carrots, celery and green pepper in a large Dutch oven or soup kettle. Bring to a boil; reduce heat and simmer for 20 minutes or until vegetables are soft. Cool. Press mixture through a food mill or fine sieve. Return juice to Dutch oven; add sugar, Worcestershire sauce and pepper. Bring to a boil.

Ladle hot juice into hot sterilized quart jars, leaving 1/4-in. headspace. Add 2 tablespoons lemon juice to each jar. Adjust caps. Process for 40 minutes in a boiling-water bath. **Yield:** 7-8 quarts.

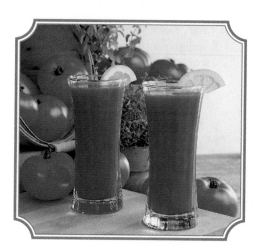

Exchanges: 2 Vegetable

Nutritional Information

Serving Size: 1/2 cup
Calories: 46
Sodium: 15 mg
Cholesterol: 0

Carbohydrate: 10 gm
Protein: 2 gm
Fat: trace

Triple Cheese Spread

Debbi Smith, Crossett, Arkansas

Even folks not on restricted diets will love this cheesy and creamy spread. The carrots add nice color and crunch, while the combination of cheeses gives great flavor.

1 cup fat-free cottage cheese
1/2 cup shredded low-fat Swiss cheese
1/4 cup grated Parmesan cheese
2 tablespoons skim milk
1/8 teaspoon dill weed
1/8 teaspoon pepper
1/4 cup shredded carrots

In a blender or food processor, combine cheeses, milk, dill and pepper. Process until smooth. Stir in carrots. Cover and chill. Serve with crackers. **Yield:** 1-3/4 cups.

FRESH ADVICE. Cottage cheese will stay fresher longer if you store it upside down in the refrigerator.

Exchanges: 1/2 Meat
Nutritional Information

Serving Size: 2 tablespoons
Calories: 41
Sodium: 116 mg
Cholesterol: 6 mg

Carbohydrate: 1 gm
Protein: 5 gm
Fat: 2 gm

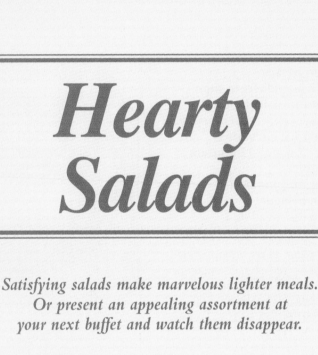

Hearty Salads

Satisfying salads make marvelous lighter meals.
Or present an appealing assortment at
your next buffet and watch them disappear.

Layered Crab Salad

Betty Nichols, Eugene, Oregon

I love living in Oregon and enjoy cooking with the many foods available in this part of the country. Crabmeat is abundant here and makes a great company dinner. I especially like it in this salad.

4 cups torn lettuce
2 cups (1/2 pound) fresh snow
  peas, cut into 1-inch pieces
1-1/2 cups chopped sweet red pepper
2 cups chopped cucumber
1 package (8 ounces) imitation
  crabmeat
1 cup light mayonnaise
1 tablespoon sugar
1 teaspoon dill weed *or* 1
  tablespoon chopped fresh dill

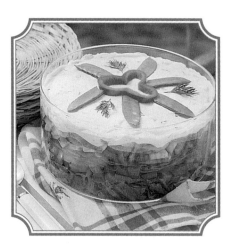

In a 2-1/2-qt. clear glass serving bowl, layer lettuce, peas, red pepper, cucumber and crab. Combine mayonnaise, sugar and dill; spread over crab. Cover and chill several hours or overnight. **Yield:** 6 servings.

Exchanges: 2 Vegetable, 1 Meat, 1 Fat
Nutritional Information

Serving Size: 1/6 recipe
Calories: 180
Sodium: 579 mg
Cholesterol: 16 mg

Carbohydrate: 13 gm
Protein: 8 gm
Fat: 11 gm

Sesame Beef and Asparagus Salad

Tamara Steeb, Issaquah, Washington

Especially during the summer, this makes a nice light meal. It's quick and easy, but it always wins me many compliments. Cooking is one of my favorite hobbies…I like to experiment with different recipes.

1 pound top round steak
4 cups sliced fresh asparagus
(2-inch pieces)
3 tablespoons light soy sauce
2 tablespoons sesame oil
1 tablespoon rice wine vinegar
1/2 teaspoon grated gingerroot
Sesame seeds
Lettuce leaves, optional

Broil steak to desired doneness. Cool and cut into thin diagonal strips. Cook asparagus in a small amount of water 30-60 seconds. Drain and cool. Combine beef and asparagus. Blend all remaining ingredients except the last two; pour over beef and asparagus. Sprinkle with sesame seeds and toss lightly. Serve warm or at room temperature, on lettuce if desired. **Yield:** 6 servings.

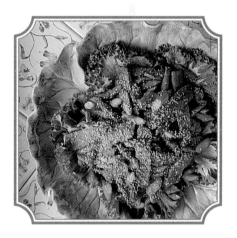

Exchanges: 2 Lean Meat, 1-1/2 Vegetable, 1/2 Fat

Nutritional Information

Serving Size: 1/6 recipe
Calories: 179
Sodium: 366 mg
Cholesterol: 48 mg

Carbohydrate: 6 gm
Protein: 21 gm
Fat: 8 gm

Hot Chicken Salad

Michelle Wise, Spring Mills, Pennsylvania

This simple yet delicious recipe originated with my aunt and was passed on to my mom. It's great for a luncheon...or, served with salad and rolls, for supper. With three children, I need all the fast dishes I can find!

2-1/2 cups diced cooked chicken breast
   1 cup diced celery
   1 cup sliced fresh mushrooms
   1 tablespoon minced onion
   1 teaspoon lemon juice
1/2 teaspoon dried rosemary, crushed
1/4 teaspoon pepper
   1 can (8 ounces) sliced water chestnuts, drained
   2 cups cooked rice

3/4 cup light mayonnaise
   1 can (10-3/4 ounces) condensed low-fat low-sodium cream of chicken soup, undiluted

In a 2-1/2-qt. casserole, combine first nine ingredients. Blend mayonnaise and soup; toss with chicken mixture. Spoon into a 2-qt. casserole coated with non-stick cooking spray. Bake, uncovered, at 350° for 30 minutes. **Yield:** 6 servings.

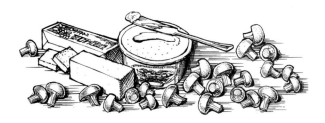

Exchanges: 2 Starch, 1 Lean Meat, 1 Vegetable, 1 Fat

Nutritional Information

Serving Size: 1/6 recipe
Calories: 265
Sodium: 305 mg
Cholesterol: 41 mg

Carbohydrate: 31 gm
Protein: 13 gm
Fat: 10 gm

Southwestern Bean Salad

Lila Jean Allen, Portland, Oregon

My daughter gave me the recipe for this hearty, zippy salad. I've used it many times and received compliments. When it comes to bean salad, most people think of the sweet three-bean variety, so this is a nice surprise.

1 can (15 to 16 ounces) kidney
  beans, rinsed and drained
1 can (15 ounces) black beans,
  rinsed and drained
1 can (15-1/2 ounces) garbanzo
  beans, rinsed and drained
2 celery ribs, sliced
1 medium red onion, diced
1 medium tomato, diced
1 cup frozen corn, thawed
DRESSING:
  3/4 cup thick and chunky salsa
  1/4 cup vegetable oil
  1/4 cup lime juice
1-1/2 teaspoons chili powder
  1/2 teaspoon ground cumin

In a bowl, combine beans, celery, onion, tomato and corn. In a small bowl, combine dressing ingredients; mix well. Pour over the bean mixture and toss to coat. Cover and chill for at least 2 hours. **Yield:** 10 servings.

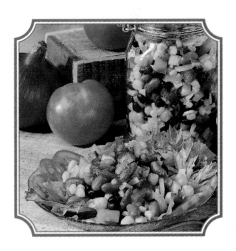

Exchanges: 2 Starch, 1 Vegetable, 1 Fat

Nutritional Information

Serving Size: 3/4 cup
Calories: 210
Sodium: 382 mg
Cholesterol: 0

Carbohydrate: 32 gm
Protein: 8 gm
Fat: 7 gm

Shrimp Pasta Salad

Sherri Gentry, Dallas, Oregon

When I'm planning a special luncheon, this pasta salad is sure to appear on the menu. This refreshing salad stirs up quickly, yet looks elegant. So it's an easy way to impress guests.

12 ounces spiral pasta, cooked and drained
1 package (10 ounces) frozen cooked shrimp, thawed
1/4 cup sliced green onions
1/4 cup grated Parmesan cheese
1/3 cup vegetable oil
1/3 cup red wine vinegar
2-1/2 teaspoons dill weed
3/4 teaspoon garlic powder
1/2 teaspoon pepper

In a large bowl, combine pasta, shrimp, onions and Parmesan cheese. In a small bowl, combine remaining ingredients. Pour over pasta mixture and toss. Cover and chill for 1-2 hours. **Yield:** 10 servings.

PERFECT PASTA . Your pasta will turn out wonderfully every time if you cook it uncovered at a fast boil. A rapid boil helps circulate the pasta for consistent results. Also be sure to stir frequently. As soon as the required cooking time has elapsed, drain the pasta to prevent further cooking.

Exchanges: 1-1/2 Starch, 1 Meat, 1/2 Vegetable, 1/2 Fat

Nutritional Information

Serving Size: 1 cup
Calories: 231
Sodium: 39 mg
Cholesterol: 45 mg

Carbohydrate: 27 gm
Protein: 12 gm
Fat: 8 gm

Pork and Spinach Salad

Marian Platt, Sequim, Washington

I serve this hearty main-dish salad at family gatherings throughout the year.
You just can't beat a salad that tastes great and is good for you, too.

10 ounces fresh spinach, washed
  and stems removed
1 can (16 ounces) black-eyed
  peas, rinsed and drained
1/3 cup low-fat Italian dressing
1/4 cup sliced green onions
1/2 cup sliced fresh mushrooms
1/4 cup sliced celery
1 jar (2 ounces) sliced pimientos,
  drained
3 tablespoons sliced ripe olives
2 garlic cloves, minced
1 tablespoon olive oil
1/2 pound pork tenderloin, cut into
  thin strips

Line four plates with spinach leaves; set aside. In a bowl, combine peas, Italian dressing, green onions, mushrooms, celery, pimientos and olives; set aside. In a medium skillet, saute garlic in oil for 30 seconds. Add pork and stir-fry for 2-3 minutes or until no pink remains. Remove from the heat; add vegetable mixture and mix well. Divide among spinach-lined plates. Serve immediately. **Yield:** 4 servings.

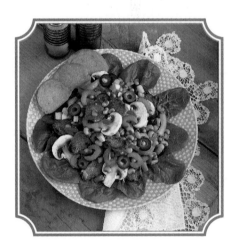

Exchanges: 3 Vegetable, 2 oz. Meat, 1 Starch, 1 Fat

Nutritional Information

Serving Size: 1/4 recipe
Calories: 317
Sodium: 758 mg
Cholesterol: 56 mg

Carbohydrate: 24 gm
Protein: 27 gm
Fat: 13 gm

My Favorite Rice Salad

Vera Melvin, St. Ann, Missouri

This rice salad came from my mother's personal cookbook. I like to make this salad for special occasions. It tastes especially good with barbecued meats and turkey dishes...and it's nutritious!

4 cups hot cooked rice
1 can (8-3/4 ounces) kidney beans, rinsed and drained
1 small onion, chopped
1/4 cup vegetable oil
2 tablespoons white vinegar
1 tablespoon sugar
1 tablespoon pickle relish
1-1/2 teaspoons chili powder
1 medium green pepper, chopped

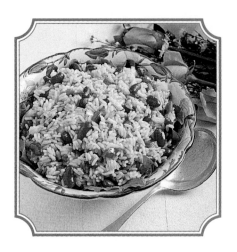

Combine rice, beans and onion. In a separate bowl, combine oil, vinegar, sugar, relish and chili powder. Toss with rice mixture. Cover and chill for several hours. Just before serving, stir in green pepper. **Yield:** 8 servings.

Exchanges: 2 Starch, 1-1/2 Fat, 1 Vegetable

Nutritional Information

Serving Size: 1/8 recipe
Calories: 239
Sodium: 201 mg
Cholesterol: 0

Carbohydrate: 40 gm
Protein: 4 gm
Fat: 7 gm

Hot Beef and Hazelnut Salad

Ruth Gooding, Los Angeles, California

In my kitchen, leftover roast frequently ends up in this filling salad.

**1 pound sirloin steak, sliced
into thin strips**
MARINADE:
  1/4 cup sliced green onions
  2 garlic cloves, minced
  2 tablespoons light soy sauce
  1 tablespoon vegetable oil
  1 tablespoon water
DRESSING:
  2 tablespoons cider vinegar
  2 tablespoons light soy sauce
  2 tablespoons vegetable oil
  1 garlic clove, minced
  1 teaspoon sugar
  1/4 teaspoon curry powder
  1/4 teaspoon ground ginger

  8 to 10 cups torn salad greens
  **1/4 cup coarsely chopped
    hazelnuts, toasted**
Sliced green onions
Chopped green *or* sweet red peppers

Place beef in a glass bowl. Combine marinade ingredients; pour over beef.

Chill 30 minutes. Meanwhile, combine dressing ingredients; set aside. Place greens in a large salad bowl; refrigerate. In a skillet over high heat, cook half the beef and marinade to desired doneness. Remove and then cook remaining beef. Drain and add all beef to greens. In the same skillet, heat dressing. Pour over salad and quickly toss. Top with hazelnuts, onions and peppers. Serve immediately. **Yield:** 4 servings.

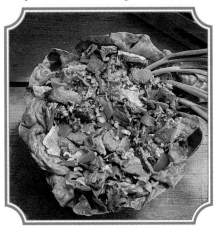

Exchanges: 3-1/2 Meat, 1 Vegetable, 1 Fat
Nutritional Information

Serving Size: 1/4 recipe
Calories: 329
Sodium: 423 mg
Cholesterol: 70 mg

Carbohydrate: 6 gm
Protein: 28 gm
Fat: 22 gm

Stir-Fry Spinach Salad

Victoria Schreur, Lowell, Michigan

I first served this at a party…it was an instant hit. I'm sure you and your family will like the slightly sweet-and-sour sauce in this unique salad.

1 can (8 ounces) pineapple chunks in natural juices
1 pound boneless skinless chicken breasts, julienned
2 tablespoons cooking oil
1 medium green pepper, julienned
3 tablespoons brown sugar
1 tablespoon cornstarch
1/4 cup ketchup
3 tablespoons vinegar
2 tablespoons light soy sauce
6 cups torn fresh spinach
1 cup cherry tomato halves

Drain pineapple, reserving 3 tablespoons juice in a small bowl; set the pineapple aside. (Discard remaining juice or save for another use.) In a skillet or wok, stir-fry chicken in oil for 5 minutes or until no longer pink. Add green pepper; stir-fry for 2-4 minutes or until crisp-tender. Meanwhile, add brown sugar and cornstarch to pineapple juice; mix well. Stir in ketchup, vinegar and soy sauce until smooth; add to skillet and cook until thickened. On a large serving platter, arrange spinach, pineapple and tomatoes. Top with chicken and green pepper; serve immediately. **Yield:** 6 servings.

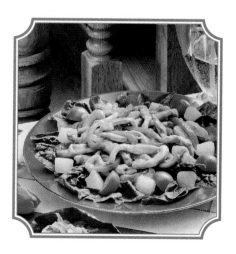

Exchanges: 2 Lean Meat, 2 Vegetable, 1 Fruit
Nutritional Information

Serving Size: 1/6 recipe
Calories: 230
Sodium: 480 mg
Cholesterol: 53 mg

Carbohydrate: 22 gm
Protein: 21 gm
Fat: 8 gm

Tuna Egg Salad

Daisy Brocato, Raceland, Louisiana

People can't believe it when I tell them this recipe does fit into a diet-restricted menu. Everyone loves the old-fashioned flavor of this tasty traditional tuna salad.

1 hard-cooked egg, chopped
1 can (3 ounces) light tuna in
   spring water, drained and flaked
1/4 cup chopped celery
1/4 cup chopped sweet pickles
3 tablespoons light mayonnaise
2 teaspoons prepared mustard

Combine all of the ingredients in a small bowl and mix well. Spoon into tomatoes, use as a sandwich filling or serve with crackers. **Yield:** 3 servings (1-1/4 cups).

"EGGS-CELLENT" TIPS.

Crack cooked shells slightly. Let stand in cold water 5 minutes and then peel.

If you dip a knife in water before slicing hard-cooked eggs, the eggs won't crumble.

To prevent dark surfaces on yolks of hard-cooked eggs, immediately run cold water over the cooked eggs or place them in ice water until completely cooled.

Hard-cooked eggs can be stored in the refrigerator for up to 1 week.

Exchanges: 1-1/2 Meat, 1 Vegetable

Nutritional Information

Serving Size: 1/3 recipe
Calories: 129
Sodium: 396 mg
Cholesterol: 86 mg

Carbohydrate: 7 gm
Protein: 11 gm
Fat: 6 gm

Curried Chicken Salad

Tina Krasicki, Decatur, Illinois

I usually serve this salad on a big lettuce leaf with breadsticks and fresh melon wedges. However you serve it, no one will be able to resist the terrific combination of tasty chicken, sweet fruit and crunchy almonds.

3 cups diced cooked chicken
1/2 cup finely chopped celery
1 can (8 ounces) water
  chestnuts, drained
1 medium apple, cored and diced
3/4 cup halved green grapes
1 can (8 ounces) pineapple
  tidbits in natural juices, juice
  drained and reserved
1/2 cup raisins
1/2 cup slivered almonds
DRESSING:
1-1/4 cups light mayonnaise
1/4 cup reserved pineapple juice
1 tablespoon light soy sauce
1 tablespoon vinegar
1/4 teaspoon lemon *or* lime juice
1 to 3 teaspoons curry powder

In a large bowl, combine first eight ingredients. Blend all dressing ingredients and toss with chicken mixture. Chill several hours. **Yield:** 8 servings.

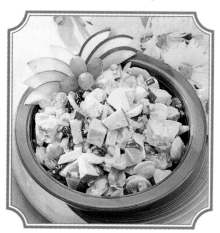

Exchanges: 2-1/2 Lean Meat, 1-1/2 Fruit, 1 Vegetable, 1 Fat

Nutritional Information

Serving Size: 1/8 recipe
Calories: 297
Sodium: 348 mg
Cholesterol: 96 mg

Carbohydrate: 30 gm
Protein: 18 gm
Fat: 12 gm

Country Rice Salad

Arlyn Kramer, El Campo, Texas

This recipe makes a nice change from potato salad, and it goes well with any main meal. A lot of rice is grown here in Wharton County, and this is a delicious way to prepare it.

DRESSING:
- 1/2 cup light mayonnaise
- 1/4 cup prepared mustard
- 2 tablespoons sugar
- 1 teaspoon vinegar
- 1/4 teaspoon salt
- 1/8 teaspoon pepper
- 1 to 2 tablespoons skim milk, if necessary

SALAD:
- 3 cups cooked rice, chilled
- 1/4 cup sweet pickle relish
- 1 jar (2 ounces) chopped pimientos, drained
- 1/3 cup finely chopped green onions (including tops)
- 1/4 cup finely chopped green pepper
- 1/4 cup finely chopped celery
- 3 hard-cooked eggs, diced

Combine all dressing ingredients except the milk. Set aside. In a large salad bowl, combine first seven salad ingredients. Add dressing; stir gently. Add milk if mixture is dry. Chill several hours before serving. **Yield:** 10 servings.

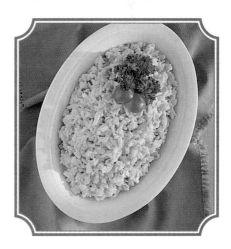

Exchanges: 1 Starch, 1 Fat, 1/2 Vegetable

Nutritional Information

Serving Size: 1/10 recipe
Calories: 144
Sodium: 280 mg
Cholesterol: 85 mg

Carbohydrate: 20 gm
Protein: 3 gm
Fat: 5 gm

Smoked Turkey and Apple Salad

Carolyn Popwell, Lacey, Washington

This eye-catching salad makes a refreshing main course for a light lunch or dinner. The dressing's Dijon flavor goes nicely with the turkey, while the apples and walnuts add crunch.

DRESSING:
- 2 tablespoons cider vinegar
- 5 tablespoons olive oil
- 1 tablespoon Dijon mustard
- 1 teaspoon lemon pepper

SALAD:
- 1 bunch romaine, torn into bite-size pieces
- 1 carrot, julienned
- 10 cherry tomatoes, halved
- 8 ounces smoked turkey, julienned
- 4 unpeeled apples, sliced
- 1/3 cup chopped walnuts, toasted

Whisk together dressing ingredients and set aside. Just before serving, arrange romaine on a platter or individual plates. Top with carrot, tomatoes, turkey and apples. Drizzle with dressing and sprinkle with walnuts. **Yield:** 8 servings.

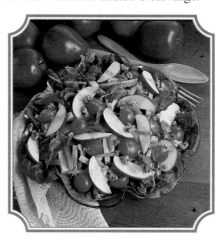

Exchanges: 2 Fat, 1-1/2 Vegetable, 1 Meat

Nutritional Information

Serving Size: 1/8 recipe
Calories: 195
Sodium: 267 mg
Cholesterol: 8 mg

Carbohydrate: 10 gm
Protein: 6 gm
Fat: 16 gm

Greek Chicken Salad

Donna Smith, Palisade, Colorado

My family loves this salad—I receive nothing but raves when I serve it. Even if you or your family are not garlic lovers, I'd advise that you use the full measurement of garlic and oregano for the proper flavoring.

3 cups cubed cooked chicken
2 medium cucumbers, peeled, seeded and chopped
1 cup crumbled feta cheese
2/3 cup sliced ripe olives
1/4 cup minced fresh parsley
1 cup light mayonnaise
3 garlic cloves, minced
1/2 cup plain yogurt
1 tablespoon dried oregano

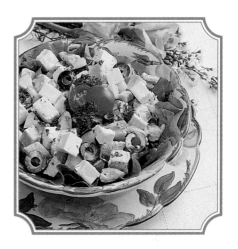

Combine the first five ingredients. Set aside. In a small bowl, combine remaining ingredients. Toss with chicken mixture. Cover and chill for several hours. **Yield:** 7 servings.

Exchanges: 2-1/2 Meat, 2 Vegetable, 1 Fat

Nutritional Information

Serving Size: 1/7 recipe
Calories: 288
Sodium: 566 mg
Cholesterol: 80 mg

Carbohydrate: 11 gm
Protein: 23 gm
Fat: 17 gm

Minty Rice Salad

Naomi Giddis, Grawn, Michigan

When my garden is at its peak, I love to prepare this refreshing salad using my own tomatoes, cucumbers, radishes, green peppers and mint. Make this wonderful dish ahead to allow the flavors to blend and for added convenience.

2 cups cooked brown rice
3 medium tomatoes, seeded and finely chopped
1 cup fresh *or* frozen peas
1 cucumber, seeded and finely chopped
1 green pepper, finely chopped
1/2 cup sliced green onions
1/2 cup sliced radishes
1/3 cup olive oil
3 tablespoons lemon juice
2 tablespoons chopped fresh mint
1/4 teaspoon pepper

In a large bowl, combine rice, tomatoes, peas, cucumber, green pepper, onions and radishes; set aside. In a small bowl, combine remaining ingredients. Pour over rice and vegetables; mix well. Chill for at least 1 hour. Serve cold. **Yield:** 6 servings.

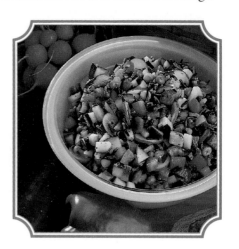

Exchanges: 2 Fat, 1-1/2 Starch, 1 Vegetable

Nutritional Information

Serving Size: 1/6 recipe
Calories: 231
Sodium: 225 mg
Cholesterol: 0

Carbohydrate: 27 gm
Protein: 5 gm
Fat: 12 gm

Grilled Chicken Salad

Virginia Pugh Moon, Harvest, Alabama

*Finding foods that my husband will eat is sometimes a challenge.
I came up with this grilled chicken salad in an effort to duplicate
one of his favorite restaurant dishes. He ate every bite!*

  1 **can (8 ounces) pineapple tidbits
     in natural juices**
  3 **tablespoons light soy sauce**
  1 **tablespoon Worcestershire sauce**
1/2 **teaspoon garlic powder**
1/4 **to 1/2 teaspoon pepper**
  2 **pounds boneless skinless
     chicken breasts, julienned**
  8 **cups torn salad greens**
  2 **large tomatoes, chopped**
  4 **green onions, sliced**

Drain pineapple, reserving juice; set pineapple aside. In a glass bowl, combine juice, soy sauce, Worcestershire sauce, garlic powder and pepper. Add chicken strips; toss to coat. Cover and chill for 2-6 hours. Grill or broil chicken strips, turning to brown both sides, for 8-10 minutes or until juices run clear. To serve, line four plates with greens; arrange tomatoes, onions, pineapple and warm chicken over greens. **Yield:** 4 servings.

A REAL CUTUP. When a recipe requires you to cut raw meat, such as chicken, partially freeze the meat beforehand. You'll find it's easier and faster to slice.

Exchanges: 6 Lean Meat, 1 Vegetable, 1/2 Fruit

Nutritional Information

Serving Size: 1/4 recipe
Calories: 383
Sodium: 381 mg
Cholesterol: 159 mg

Carbohydrate: 17 gm
Protein: 58 gm
Fat: 9 gm

Black-Eyed Pea Salad

Martha Sue Stroud, Clarksville, Texas

Each time I take this dish to a church supper, I get many requests for the recipe. It is inexpensive to make, and the red onion rings add a nice touch of color to a meal. The real beauty of this salad is that it can be made well ahead of time.

2 cans (16 ounces *each*) black-eyed peas, rinsed and drained
1/2 cup red onion rings
1/2 cup chopped green pepper
1 small garlic clove, minced
1 teaspoon sugar
1/4 cup vinegar
1/4 cup vegetable oil
Dash pepper
Dash hot pepper sauce

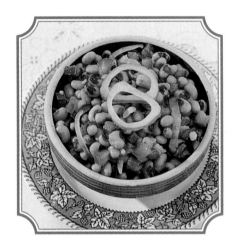

In a medium salad bowl, combine peas, onion, green pepper and garlic. Stir together all remaining ingredients and pour over vegetable mixture. Cover and chill for at least 12 hours. **Yield:** 8 servings. **Editor's Note:** Ingredients can be easily divided to prepare just half of the recipe.

Exchanges: 1-1/2 Fat, 1 Starch, 1/2 Vegetable

Nutritional Information

Serving Size: 1/8 recipe
Calories: 162
Sodium: 359 mg
Cholesterol: 0

Carbohydrate: 19 gm
Protein: 6 gm
Fat: 8 gm

Wild Rice Salad

Florence Jacoby, Granite Falls, Minnesota

Since I spend part of my summers in northern Minnesota near the wild rice fields, I have tried many recipes featuring this delicious, nutty-flavored grain. This salad is often requested by family and friends.

1 cup uncooked wild rice
2 cups diced cooked chicken
1-1/2 cups halved green grapes
1 cup sliced water chestnuts,
**   drained**
3/4 cup light mayonnaise
Lettuce leaves

Cook rice according to package directions, omitting salt. Drain well; cool to room temperature. Spoon into a large bowl; add chicken, grapes, water chestnuts and mayonnaise. Toss gently with a fork. Cover and chill. Serve on lettuce leaves or line a bowl with lettuce leaves and fill with salad. **Yield:** 6 servings.

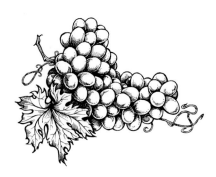

Exchanges: 2 Lean Meat, 1 Starch, 1 Fruit, 1 Vegetable, 1 Fat
Nutritional Information
Serving Size: 1/6 recipe
Calories: 318
Sodium: 229 mg
Cholesterol: 38 mg

Carbohydrate: 40 gm
Protein: 19 gm
Fat: 10 gm

Crunchy Chicken Salad

Diane Hixon, Niceville, Florida

*This special salad is packed with hearty chicken,
fresh produce and fantastic flavor. Best of all, it's good for you.
So you can enjoy every flavorful bite.*

4 cups shredded cooked
  chicken
2 cups shredded lettuce
1 cup julienned carrots
1 cup julienned cucumber
2/3 cup green onion strips (2-inch
  pieces)
1 cup fresh bean sprouts
DRESSING:
2 tablespoons vegetable oil
2 tablespoons lemon juice
2 tablespoons sesame seeds,
  toasted
1-1/2 teaspoons light soy sauce
1/4 teaspoon pepper
1/4 teaspoon dry mustard
Hot pepper sauce to taste

In a large salad bowl, toss the chicken, lettuce, carrots, cucumber, green onion and bean sprouts. Refrigerate. In a small bowl, combine dressing ingredients. Refrigerate. Just before serving, pour dressing over salad and toss gently. **Yield:** 10 servings.

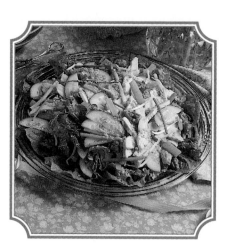

Exchanges: 2 Lean Meat, 1 Vegetable, 1/2 Fat

Nutritional Information

Serving Size: 1 cup
Calories: 156
Sodium: 201 mg
Cholesterol: 42 mg

Carbohydrate: 5 gm
Protein: 19 gm
Fat: 6 gm

Macaroni Salad with Basil Dressing

Christine Gibson, Fontana, Wisconsin

My sister and I came up with this great-tasting salad when my husband and I planned our first garden...and overdid the tomato and zucchini plants! We have our garden under control today but still make this popular dish.

1 cup loosely packed fresh basil leaves
3 garlic cloves
1/2 teaspoon pepper
2/3 cup olive oil
1 tablespoon red wine vinegar
3 medium tomatoes, seeded and diced
2 to 3 medium zucchini, cut into 1/4-inch slices
7 to 8 ounces elbow macaroni, cooked and drained
2 cups (8 ounces) shredded low-fat mozzarella cheese

In a blender container or food processor, combine the basil, garlic and pepper. Process until finely chopped. Add oil and vinegar; process until well blended. Set aside. In a 4-qt. salad bowl, combine tomatoes, zucchini, macaroni and cheese; toss lightly. Pour dressing over all; toss to coat. Cover and refrigerate at least 2 hours or overnight. **Yield:** 10 servings.

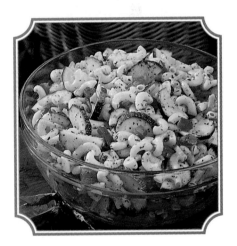

Exchanges: 3 Fat, 1 Starch, 1 Vegetable, 1 Meat

Nutritional Information

Serving Size: 1-1/4 cups
Calories: 273
Sodium: 126 mg
Cholesterol: 12 mg

Carbohydrate: 21 gm
Protein: 10 gm
Fat: 18 gm

Wild Rice and Turkey Salad

Ginny Schneider, Muenster, Texas

I prepare this colorful salad often around the holidays when leftover turkey is abundant. But you and your family will enjoy it any time of year!

4 cups torn fresh spinach
2 cups cubed cooked turkey breast
2 cups cooked wild rice
1 medium onion, chopped
1 cup sliced fresh mushrooms
2 medium tomatoes, chopped
1 jar (2 ounces) chopped
   pimientos, drained

1 bottle (8 ounces) fat-free Italian
   salad dressing

In a large bowl, combine the first seven ingredients. Add dressing just before serving; toss to coat. **Yield:** 9 servings.

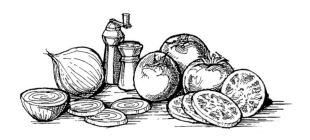

Exchanges: 1 Starch, 1 Lean Meat, 1 Vegetable

Nutritional Information

Serving Size: 1 cup
Calories: 157
Sodium: 71 mg
Cholesterol: 10 mg

Carbohydrate: 21 gm
Protein: 14 gm
Fat: 2 gm

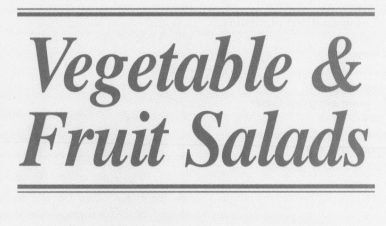

Vegetable & Fruit Salads

*Why not reach for these produce-packed
salads for a refreshing change of pace?
You're bound to harvest a bushel of smiles!*

Dilly Asparagus

Margot Foster, Hubbard, Texas

This asparagus dish has been in my recipe file so long I can't remember where it originated. It makes a good cool vegetable on a hot day.

1 pound fresh asparagus, trimmed
1 jar (2 ounces) diced pimientos, drained
1/2 cup vinegar
1/4 cup olive oil
1 tablespoon sugar
1 tablespoon chopped fresh parsley
2 teaspoons dried minced onion
1 teaspoon dill weed
1/4 teaspoon coarse ground black pepper

Cook the asparagus in a small amount of water until crisp-tender. Drain. In a jar with a tight-fitting lid, combine all the remaining ingredients and shake well. Place asparagus in a shallow dish; pour marinade over asparagus. Cover and refrigerate 8 hours. To serve, remove asparagus and arrange on a platter; remove pimientos and onion from marinade with a slotted spoon and sprinkle over asparagus. **Yield:** 4 servings.

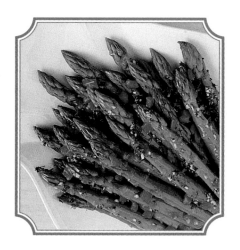

Exchanges: 2-1/2 Fat, 1 Vegetable, 1/2 Starch
Nutritional Information
Serving Size: 1/4 recipe
Calories: 173
Sodium: 33 mg
Cholesterol: 0
Carbohydrate: 11 gm
Protein: 3 gm
Fat: 14 gm

Light Potato Salad

Sharon Thom, Lavina, Montana

My husband and I are both from big families, so we're always getting together for picnics and dinners. No matter how often I serve this salad, everyone loves it.

2 pounds unpeeled red potatoes, cooked and cubed (5 cups)
1/2 cup chopped celery
1/4 cup chopped dill pickle
2 tablespoons chopped sweet red pepper
2 tablespoons chopped onion
2 tablespoons snipped fresh parsley
1-1/2 teaspoons snipped fresh mint
or 1/2 teaspoon dried mint
2 tablespoons plain low-fat yogurt
2 tablespoons lemon juice
1/2 teaspoon honey
1/4 teaspoon dry mustard
3/4 teaspoon snipped fresh basil
or 1/4 teaspoon dried basil
1/4 teaspoon pepper

In bowl, combine potatoes, celery, pickle, red pepper, onion, parsley and mint. Combine all remaining ingredients; pour over salad and mix gently. Cover and chill for several hours. **Yield:** 10 servings.

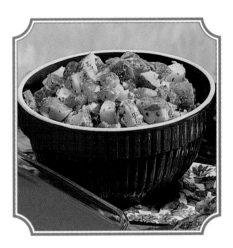

Exchanges: 1 Starch

Nutritional Information

Serving Size: 1/2 cup
Calories: 63
Sodium: 74 mg
Cholesterol: 0

Carbohydrate: 14 gm
Protein: 2 gm
Fat: trace

Orange and Red Onion Salad

Nancy Schmidt, Gustine, California

Orange and onion does sound like an unusual combination. But when my husband tasted it for the first time, he proclaimed it an instant success. I serve this refreshing salad with a variety of meats and think it goes especially well with chicken.

2 tablespoons fresh lemon juice
1 teaspoon Dijon mustard
1/2 teaspoon sugar
1/2 teaspoon salt
1/4 teaspoon white pepper
1/2 cup vegetable oil
1 bunch romaine, torn into
  bite-size pieces

2 medium oranges, peeled and
  sectioned
1 small red onion, thinly sliced

In a small bowl, combine first five ingredients. Beat in oil. Combine lettuce, oranges and onion. Toss with dressing. Serve immediately. **Yield:** 6 servings.

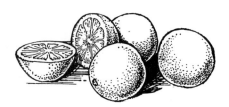

Exchanges: 3-1/2 Fat, 1 Vegetable
Nutritional Information
Serving Size: 1/6 recipe
Calories: 193
Sodium: 207 mg
Cholesterol: 0

Carbohydrate: 8 gm
Protein: 1 gm
Fat: 18 gm

Cathy's Tomato-Bean Salad

Cathy Meizel, Flanders, New York

*My mother and grandmother made this salad often...
but I eventually made some adjustments by accident. You see, one night, I was
preparing dinner for my future husband and wanted to impress him with
my cooking. But my cupboards were bare—except for a can of "chick-peas" and
one of olives. Into the salad they went. And he loved the results!*

1 can (15 ounces) garbanzo
   beans, rinsed and drained
4 large ripe tomatoes, thickly
   sliced
1 cup thinly sliced red onion
1 can (6 ounces) medium pitted
   ripe olives, drained and halved
1/2 cup olive oil
5 to 6 large fresh basil leaves,
   snipped *or* 1 tablespoon dried
   basil
1/2 teaspoon dried oregano
1/4 teaspoon pepper
1/8 teaspoon garlic powder

In a large salad bowl, layer beans, tomatoes, onion and olives. Combine all remaining ingredients; pour over vegetables. Cover and chill at least 3 hours or overnight. Serve chilled or at room temperature. **Yield:** 8 servings.

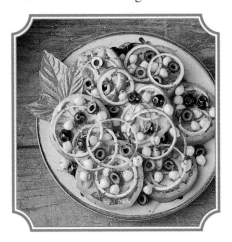

Exchanges: 2 Fat, 1 Starch, 1 Vegetable

Nutritional Information

Serving Size: 1/8 recipe
Calories: 178
Sodium: 333 mg
Cholesterol: 0

Carbohydrate: 19 gm
Protein: 4 gm
Fat: 10 gm

Carrot-Lentil Salad

Monica Wilcott, Sturgis, Saskatchewan

I got this recipe in a "swap" with one of my sisters. People usually aren't familiar with lentils, so they'll try only a little at first. Before long, though, they'll ask for a "real" helping! I've found this is an ideal dish to take out to the field.

1 cup dry lentils
1 cup diced carrots
2 garlic cloves, minced
1 bay leaf
DRESSING:
  1/2 cup finely chopped celery
  1/4 cup finely chopped fresh
    parsley
  1/4 cup olive oil
  1/4 cup lemon juice
  1 teaspoon salt
  1/2 teaspoon dried thyme
  1/4 teaspoon pepper

In a Dutch oven, combine lentils, carrots, garlic and bay leaf. Cover with 1 in. of water. Bring to a boil, then simmer 15-20 minutes or until lentils are tender. Remove bay leaf; drain and cool. Meanwhile, combine all dressing ingredients. Pour over lentil mixture. Cover and refrigerate several hours. **Yield:** 6 servings.

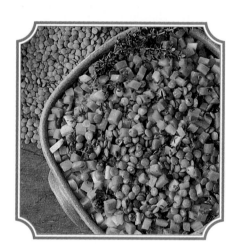

Exchanges: 2 Fat, 1-1/2 Vegetable, 1 Starch
Nutritional Information

Serving Size: 1/6 recipe
Calories: 202
Sodium: 403 mg
Cholesterol: 0

Carbohydrate: 23 gm
Protein: 8 gm
Fat: 9 gm

Zucchini Coleslaw

Aloma Hawkins, Bixby, Missouri

This salad is a treat for the eyes and the taste buds. Guests always comment on how good it looks, and I'm glad to serve a dish that's attractive. But looks don't count for much if a dish doesn't taste good, too.

2 cups coarsely shredded zucchini
2 cups shredded cabbage
1 medium carrot, shredded
2 green onions, sliced
1/2 cup thinly sliced radishes
1/3 cup light mayonnaise
1/3 cup mild picante sauce
1/2 teaspoon ground cumin

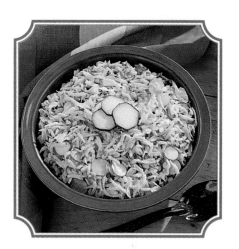

Drain zucchini by pressing between layers of paper towels. Place in a large bowl; add cabbage, carrot, onions and radishes. In a small bowl, combine remaining ingredients. Pour over vegetables and toss well. Cover and chill at least 1 hour. **Yield:** 8 servings.

Exchanges: 1 Vegetable, 1/2 Fat

Nutritional Information

Serving Size: 1/8 recipe
Calories: 55
Sodium: 154 mg
Cholesterol: 2 mg

Carbohydrate: 7 gm
Protein: 1 gm
Fat: 3 gm

Tomato Asparagus Salad

Ruby Williams, Bogalusa, Louisiana

Here's a light yet satisfying salad you're sure to enjoy all summer long. The zesty Italian dressing really enhances the fantastic flavor of refreshing produce. Even folks who aren't fond of asparagus will ask for this recipe.

1 pound fresh asparagus, trimmed
4 romaine leaves
4 cups torn romaine
10 cherry tomatoes, halved
1/3 cup fat-free Italian salad
   dressing
2 tablespoons grated Parmesan
   cheese

In a large saucepan, cook asparagus in boiling water for 5-6 minutes or until crisp-tender. Place in ice water to stop cooking. Line an 11-in. x 7-in. x 2-in. pan with romaine leaves. Top with torn romaine. Drain asparagus and arrange over the romaine; top with tomatoes. Pour dressing over all. Sprinkle with cheese. Chill for 1 hour. **Yield:** 6 servings.

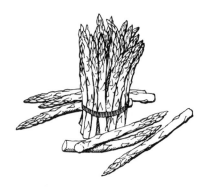

Exchanges: 2 Vegetable
Nutritional Information

Serving Size: 1/6 recipe
Calories: 62
Sodium: 174 mg
Cholesterol: 1 mg

Carbohydrate: 11 gm
Protein: 4 gm
Fat: 2 gm

Sour Cream Cucumber Salad

Lydia Robotewskyj, Franklin, Wisconsin

*This combination of sour cream and cucumbers makes a very tasty salad.
In summer, we use cucumbers from our garden for that wonderfully fresh taste.
But store-bought cucumbers work just as well, so we enjoy this dish year-round.*

3 medium cucumbers, peeled
   and thinly sliced
1/2 teaspoon salt
1/2 cup finely chopped green
   onions
1 tablespoon white vinegar
Dash white pepper
1/4 cup light sour cream

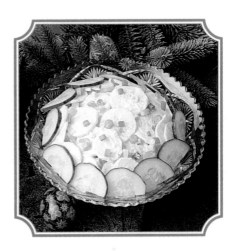

Sprinkle the cucumbers with salt. Let
stand 15 minutes. Drain liquid. Add onions, vinegar and pepper. Just before serving, stir in sour cream. **Yield:** 6 servings.

DON'T TOSS OUT a cucumber that has begun to
soften. It can be made crisp again by slicing it and
placing in ice water. Let stand 30 minutes or so, drain
and pat dry on paper towels.

Exchanges: 1 Vegetable
Nutritional Information

Serving Size: 1/6 recipe   Carbohydrate: 6 gm
Calories: 35   Protein: 2 gm
Sodium: 197 mg   Fat: 1 gm
Cholesterol: 2 mg

Sweet Potato Salad

Lettie Baker, Pennsboro, West Virginia

When I took this salad to a potluck dinner, several people asked me for the recipe. The sweet potatoes make it unique, and it really is delicious. I think you'll agree it's a nice change of pace from traditional potato salads.

3 pounds sweet potatoes, cooked,
   peeled and cubed
1/2 cup finely chopped onion
1 cup chopped green pepper
1/4 teaspoon pepper
1-1/2 cups light mayonnaise
Dash hot pepper sauce

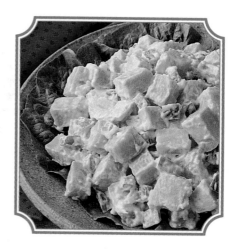

Combine first four ingredients in a large bowl. Stir in mayonnaise and hot pepper sauce; mix well. Cover and refrigerate at least 1 hour before serving. **Yield:** 10 servings.

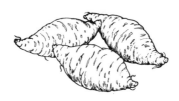

Exchanges: 2 Starch, 1-1/2 Fat

Nutritional Information

Serving Size: 1/10 recipe
Calories: 217
Sodium: 167 mg
Cholesterol: 5 mg

Carbohydrate: 38 gm
Protein: 4 gm
Fat: 7 gm

Asparagus and Tomato Salad

Nanci Brewer, San Jose, California

I created this recipe years ago. I wanted to serve a cold dish in place of a hot vegetable at a dinner we were having. I've found most everyone likes asparagus prepared this way.

1/4 cup water
1/4 teaspoon onion powder
  1 pound fresh asparagus,
    trimmed
  8 to 16 lettuce leaves
  2 to 3 large tomatoes, sliced
  1 ripe avocado, sliced
DRESSING:
  1/2 cup fat-free mayonnaise
  1/2 cup fat-free sour cream
    2 teaspoons prepared mustard
    1 teaspoon ketchup
Pepper to taste

Combine the water and onion powder; bring to a boil. Add the asparagus and cook 3-5 minutes or until asparagus is crisp-tender and bright green. Drain; cool to room temperature. Place 1-2 lettuce leaves per serving on a large platter or individual salad plates. Halve the tomato slices and arrange over lettuce. Top tomatoes with spears of asparagus and slices of avocado if desired. Combine all dressing ingredients; top each serving with a generous dollop. **Yield:** 8 servings.

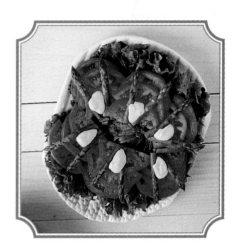

Exchanges: 1-1/2 Vegetable, 1 Fat
Nutritional Information

Serving Size: 1/8 salad recipe
with 2 tablespoons dressing
Calories: 96
Sodium: 134 mg

Cholesterol: 9 mg
Carbohydrate: 9 gm
Protein: 3 gm
Fat: 4 gm

Zucchini Harvest Salad

Marie Wellman, Seattle, Washington

Like everyone, I'm always looking for new recipes for this versatile abundant vegetable. This dish is easy to prepare, stores well and is colorful. You'll find this salad goes well with pork and chicken.

4 cups thinly sliced zucchini
1 cup sliced celery
1/2 cup sliced fresh mushrooms
1/2 cup sliced ripe olives
1/4 cup chopped green pepper
1/4 cup chopped sweet red pepper
1 cup picante sauce *or* salsa
1/2 cup vinegar
3 tablespoons olive oil
3 tablespoons sugar
1/2 teaspoon oregano
1 garlic clove, minced
Lettuce leaves

In a large bowl, combine first six ingredients; toss to mix. In a small bowl or jar, combine all remaining ingredients except lettuce and shake or mix well. Pour over vegetables. Cover and chill several hours or overnight. Serve in a large salad bowl lined with lettuce or in individual lettuce "cups". **Yield:** 8 servings.

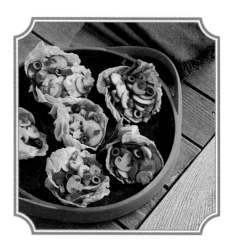

Exchanges: 1-1/2 Vegetable, 1-1/2 Fat

Nutritional Information

Serving Size: 1/8 recipe
Calories: 113
Sodium: 37 mg
Cholesterol: 0

Carbohydrate: 13 gm
Protein: 2 gm
Fat: 7 gm

Low-Fat Potato Salad

Paula Pelis, Rocky Point, New York
(ALSO PICTURED ON FRONT COVER)

Everyone in my family looks forward to hearty potato salad throughout the summer. But I want to watch my calorie intake. So I was thrilled to find the recipe for this crunchy, refreshing low-fat version.

1-1/2 pounds small salad potatoes
3/4 cup plain fat-free yogurt
3 tablespoons white wine vinegar
1 tablespoon minced fresh dill
1 tablespoon minced fresh parsley
2 teaspoons minced fresh tarragon
1/2 medium onion, chopped
1 celery rib, chopped
1 small carrot, coarsely shredded

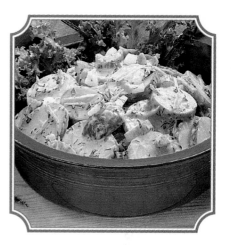

Cook potatoes until tender but firm; cool and slice. In a large bowl, combine remaining ingredients. Add potatoes and stir until well coated. Chill for several hours. **Yield:** 8 servings.

Exchanges: 1 Starch
Nutritional Information

Serving Size: 1/8 recipe
Calories: 78
Sodium: 19 mg
Cholesterol: trace

Carbohydrate: 17 gm
Protein: 3 gm
Fat: trace

Marinated Tomatoes

Myrtle Matthews, Marietta, Georgia

My niece introduced me to this colorful recipe some time ago. I now make it when I have buffets or large gatherings because it can be prepared hours ahead. This is a great way to use a bumper crop of tomatoes.

3 large fresh tomatoes, thickly sliced
1/3 cup olive oil
1/4 cup red wine vinegar
1/4 teaspoon pepper
1/2 garlic clove, minced
2 tablespoons chopped onion
1 tablespoon chopped fresh parsley
1 tablespoon chopped fresh basil *or* 1 teaspoon dried basil

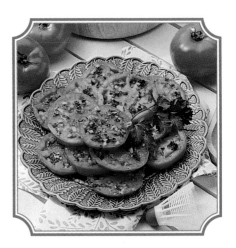

Arrange tomatoes in a large shallow dish. Combine remaining ingredients in a jar; cover tightly and shake well. Pour over tomato slices. Cover and refrigerate for several hours. **Yield:** 8 servings.

Exchanges: 2 Fat, 1/2 Vegetable
Nutritional Information

Serving Size: 1/8 recipe
Calories: 91
Sodium: 6 mg
Cholesterol: 0

Carbohydrate: 3 gm
Protein: 1 gm
Fat: 9 gm

Turnip Slaw

Vera Wiesmeur, Cove, Arkansas

*I found this recipe in a local newspaper almost 20 years ago.
I'd never heard of slaw made from turnips, but I tried it.
My husband loves it better than any cabbage slaw.*

1/4 cup chopped sweet red pepper
1/4 cup thinly sliced green onions
1/4 cup light mayonnaise
1 tablespoon vinegar
2 tablespoons sugar
1/4 teaspoon salt
1/4 teaspoon pepper
4 cups shredded peeled turnips

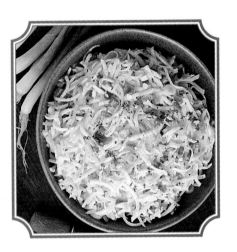

In a bowl, combine all ingredients except turnips. Pour over turnips and toss well to coat. Refrigerate several hours for flavors to blend. **Yield:** 4 servings.

ODOR EATER. Placing a charcoal briquette in a bowl in the refrigerator quickly eliminates the odor of items like onions.

Exchanges: 2 Vegetable, 1 Fat

Nutritional Information

Serving Size: 1/4 recipe
Calories: 113
Sodium: 305 mg
Cholesterol: 6 mg

Carbohydrate: 18 gm
Protein: 2 gm
Fat: 4 gm

Spicy Citrus Salad

Susan Seymour, Valatie, New York

Cooking is a favorite hobby of mine. Everyone jokes about my numerous cookbooks and five recipe boxes! I'm always looking for something new, so when I received this recipe from my nephew's wife, I had to try it.

1/2 teaspoon cayenne pepper
1 teaspoon paprika
1/2 teaspoon garlic powder
3 tablespoons olive oil
1 tablespoon wine vinegar
3 large seedless oranges,
   peeled and sectioned
1/3 cup chopped fresh parsley
18 pitted ripe olives, halved
   lengthwise
1-1/2 quarts torn mixed greens

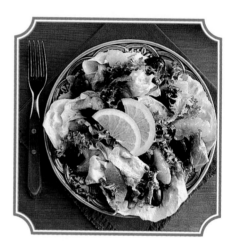

In a bowl, whisk together the first five ingredients. Stir in the oranges, parsley and olives; refrigerate 1 hour. Toss with greens and serve immediately. **Yield:** 6 servings.

Exchanges: 1 Fruit, 1 Fat, 1/2 Vegetable

Nutritional Information

Serving Size: 1/6 recipe
Calories: 112
Sodium: 114 mg
Cholesterol: 0

Carbohydrate: 15 gm
Protein: 2 gm
Fat: 6 gm

Greens with Blue Cheese Dressing

Peggy Hughes, Albany, Kentucky

*I like to make this dish with whatever greens are in season. In spring,
I use tender young greens from my own garden. It's perfect for potlucks—
just toss the dressing with the vegetables right before serving.*

1 small head cauliflower,
   broken into florets
2 quarts mixed salad greens
4 slices red onion, separated
   into rings
1/4 cup sliced stuffed olives
BLUE CHEESE DRESSING:
   2 ounces blue cheese, crumbled
1/3 cup vegetable oil
   2 tablespoons lemon juice
1/2 teaspoon sugar
1/4 teaspoon salt
   2 tablespoons chopped fresh
      parsley
   3 tablespoons chopped green
      onions

In large salad bowl, combine the first
four ingredients. Chill. Combine dressing
ingredients; toss with greens mixture just
before serving. **Yield:** 8 servings.

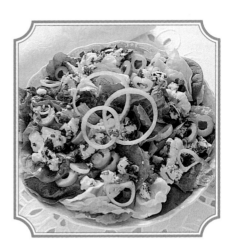

Exchanges: 2 Vegetable, 2 Fat, 1/2 Meat
Nutritional Information

Serving Size: 1/8 recipe
Calories: 181
Sodium: 310 mg
Cholesterol: 5 mg

Carbohydrate: 9 gm
Protein: 6 gm
Fat: 13 gm

Overnight Pepper Salad

Jennifer Mottashed, Simcoe, Ontario

You can pep up all sorts of events with this pretty salad. It's easy on the cook, too. Not only is it ideal for mixing up ahead of time, it can be sized right for any gathering.

1 medium green pepper, julienned
1 medium sweet red pepper, julienned
1 medium sweet yellow pepper, julienned
1 medium purple pepper, julienned
1 small red onion, julienned
1/3 cup vinegar
1/4 cup vegetable oil
1 tablespoon sugar
1 tablespoon minced fresh basil *or* 1 teaspoon dried basil
Dash pepper

In a large bowl, combine peppers and onion. Combine remaining ingredients; mix well and pour over vegetables. Cover and refrigerate 6 hours or overnight. **Yield:** 10 servings.

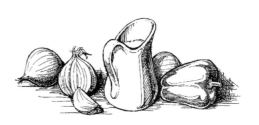

PEPPER PURCHASE. When selecting green and sweet red peppers, they should be firm and brightly colored. Refrigerate and use within 3 days.

Exchanges: 1 Fat, 1 Vegetable
Nutritional Information

Serving Size: 1/2 cup
Calories: 68
Sodium: 1 mg
Cholesterol: 0

Carbohydrate: 5 gm
Protein: 1 gm
Fat: 6 gm

Fresh Corn Salad

Carol Shaffer, Cape Girardeau, Missouri

People who prefer food with some tang find this corn salad particularly appealing. It's a pretty dish besides—and very economical.

**8 ears fresh corn, husked and
    cleaned**
1/2 cup vegetable oil
1/4 cup cider vinegar
1-1/2 teaspoons lemon juice
1/4 cup minced fresh parsley
2 teaspoons sugar
1/2 teaspoon dried basil
**1/8 to 1/4 teaspoon cayenne
    pepper**
**2 large tomatoes, seeded and
    coarsely chopped**
1/2 cup chopped onion
1/3 cup chopped green pepper
1/3 cup chopped sweet red pepper

In a large saucepan, cook corn in boiling water for 5-7 minutes or until tender. Drain, cool and set aside. In a large bowl, mix the oil, vinegar, lemon juice, parsley, sugar, basil and cayenne pepper. Cut cooled corn off the cob (should measure 4 cups). Add corn, tomatoes, onion and peppers to the oil mixture. Mix well. Cover and chill for several hours or overnight. **Yield:** 10 servings.

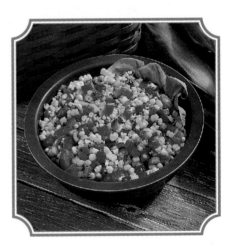

Exchanges: 1 Starch, 1/2 Vegetable, 1/2 Fat
Nutritional Information
Serving Size: 1/10 recipe
Calories: 102
Sodium: 251 mg
Cholesterol: 0

Carbohydrate: 21 gm
Protein: 3 gm
Fat: 2 gm

Spicy Coleslaw

Valerie Jones, Portland, Maine

This coleslaw is great for cookouts, group outings or anytime you want to add some spice to your menu. The green peppers and onions really bring this dish to life—and it's good for you, too. Get ready to watch it disappear!

6 cups shredded cabbage
1 cup chopped unpeeled
  cucumber
1 cup chopped tomato
1 cup chopped green pepper
1 cup sliced green onions
2/3 cup spicy V-8
1/4 cup red wine vinegar
2 teaspoons sugar
1 teaspoon celery seed
1/2 teaspoon pepper

In a large bowl, combine cabbage, cucumber, tomato, green pepper and green onions; set aside. In a small bowl, combine remaining ingredients; mix well. Pour over cabbage mixture and toss gently. Cover and chill for 2 hours; stir before serving. **Yield:** 12 servings.

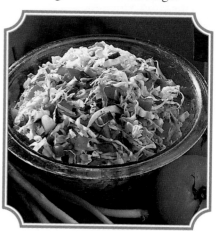

Exchanges: 1 Vegetable
Nutritional Information

Serving Size: 3/4 cup
Calories: 26
Sodium: 105 mg
Cholesterol: 0

Carbohydrate: 5 gm
Protein: 1 gm
Fat: trace

Cauliflower Salad

Paula Pelis, Rocky Point, New York

*Everyone who tries this salad loves it! I like to make it often when
cauliflower is in season. There's nothing quite like fresh Long Island produce.*

**1 medium head cauliflower,
separated into florets**
1-1/2 cups diced carrots
1 cup sliced celery
**3/4 cup sliced green onions (with
tops)**
1/2 cup sliced radishes
**1 carton (8 ounces) plain fat-free
yogurt**
**2 tablespoons white *or* tarragon
vinegar**
1 tablespoon sugar
1 teaspoon caraway seed
1 teaspoon celery seed
1/4 teaspoon pepper

In a large bowl, toss cauliflower, carrots,
celery, green onions and radishes. Combine remaining ingredients; pour over vegetables and stir to coat. Cover and chill
for several hours. **Yield:** 12 servings.

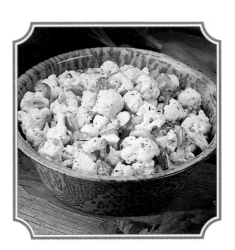

Exchanges: 1 Vegetable
Nutritional Information

Serving Size: 1/2 cup
Calories: 22
Sodium: 22 mg
Cholesterol: trace

Carbohydrate: 4 gm
Protein: 1 gm
Fat: trace

Carrot Raisin Salad

Denise Baumert, Jameson, Missouri

*This traditional salad is one of my mother-in-law's favorites.
It's fun to eat because of its crunchy texture, and the
raisins give it a slightly sweet flavor. Plus, it's easy to prepare.*

**4 cups shredded carrots (4 to 5
large)**
1 cup raisins
1/4 cup salad dressing
2 tablespoons sugar
2 to 3 tablespoons skim milk

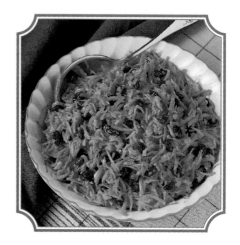

Place carrots and raisins in a bowl. In another bowl, mix together salad dressing, sugar and enough milk to reach a salad dressing consistency. Pour over carrot mixture and toss to coat. **Yield:** 8 servings.

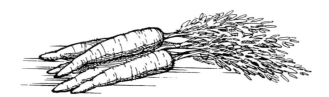

Exchanges: 1 Fruit, 1 Vegetable, 1/2 Fat
Nutritional Information

Serving Size: 1/8 recipe
Calories: 110
Sodium: 80 mg
Cholesterol: 2 mg

Carbohydrate: 24 gm
Protein: 1 gm
Fat: 2 gm

Marinated Garden Salad

Judith Anglen, Riverton, Wyoming

Not only does this colorful, tangy salad complement any main dish, it's economical besides. It uses fresh produce, so it's good for you as well.

1/2 cup sliced celery
1/2 cup sliced cucumber
1/2 cup sliced carrots
1/2 cup sliced radishes
1/2 cup light Italian salad dressing
5 cups torn salad greens

In a large bowl, combine the celery, cucumber, carrots and radishes. Add the dressing and refrigerate for 1 hour. Just before serving, add greens and toss. **Yield:** 5 servings.

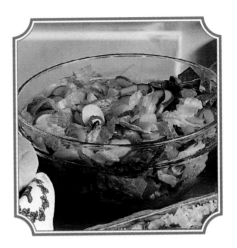

FLAVORFUL VARIATION. For a change of pace, try substituting other light dressings—like ranch or blue cheese—for the Italian salad dressing in your favorite marinated vegetable salad.

Exchanges: 1 Vegetable, 1/2 Fat

Nutritional Information

Serving Size: 1/5 recipe
Calories: 44
Sodium: 216 mg
Cholesterol: 2 mg

Carbohydrate: 5 gm
Protein: 1 gm
Fat: 3 gm

Calico Potato Salad

Christine Hartry, Emo, Ontario

One of the nice things about this salad is how versatile it is. I've taken it to potlucks, square dances...even to the field during haying season! It goes well with cold meat, like roast beef, chicken or ham.

DRESSING:
   1/2 cup olive oil
   1/4 cup vinegar
   1 tablespoon sugar
1-1/2 teaspoons chili powder
Dash hot pepper sauce
SALAD:
   4 large red potatoes (about 2
      pounds), peeled and cooked
1-1/2 cups cooked whole kernel corn
   1 cup shredded carrot
   1/2 cup chopped red onion
   1/2 cup diced green pepper
   1/2 cup diced sweet red pepper
   1/2 cup sliced ripe olives

In a small bowl or jar, combine all dressing ingredients; cover and chill. Cube potatoes; combine with corn, carrot, onion, peppers and olives in a salad bowl. Pour dressing over; toss lightly. Cover and chill. **Yield:** 14 servings.

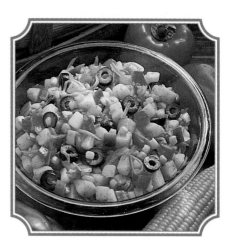

Exchanges: 1-1/2 Fat, 1 Starch
Nutritional Information

Serving Size: 1/14 recipe
Calories: 146
Sodium: 212 mg
Cholesterol: 0

Carbohydrate: 17 gm
Protein: 2 gm
Fat: 9 gm

Tomato Bread Salad

Dodi Hardcastle, Harlingen, Texas

We look forward to tomato season each year so we can make this unique and tasty recipe. It's a super dish for lunch, especially on warm summer days, and a great way to use your garden onions, cucumbers and tomatoes. It also makes a good appetizer.

3 large tomatoes, seeded and
    finely chopped
1 medium cucumber, seeded and
    finely chopped
1/2 large sweet onion, finely
    chopped
1 cup loosely packed fresh basil,
    minced
1/4 cup olive oil
1 tablespoon cider vinegar
1 garlic clove, minced
1/2 teaspoon salt
1/4 teaspoon pepper
18 slices white bread (1 inch thick)

In a large bowl, combine tomatoes, cucumber and onion. In a small bowl, combine basil, oil, vinegar, garlic, salt and pepper. Pour over tomatoes and toss. Refrigerate for at least 1 hour. Before serving, allow salad to come to room temperature. Toast bread slices under broiler until lightly browned. Top with salad. Serve immediately. **Yield:** 18 servings.

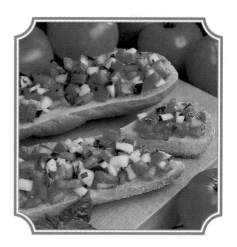

Exchanges: 1-1/2 Starch, 1 Vegetable, 1 Fat
Nutritional Information

Serving Size: 1 slice of bread
with 1/3 cup of salad
Calories: 188
Sodium: 262 mg

Cholesterol: 0
Carbohydrate: 28 gm
Protein: 5 gm
Fat: 7 gm

Quick Corn Salad

Rita Reifenstein, Evans City, Pennsylvania

This sensational salad is a delight to serve because you can make it ahead and it's an easy way to put garden bounty to good use. With colorful ingredients like corn, tomato and green pepper, it's also pretty in the bowl and on your plate.

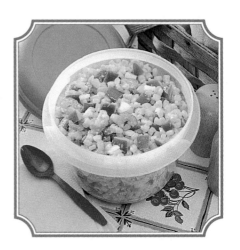

2 cups fresh *or* frozen sweet corn
3/4 cup chopped tomato
1/2 cup chopped green pepper
1/2 cup chopped celery
1/4 cup chopped onion
1/4 cup fat-free ranch salad
    dressing

In a large salad bowl, combine vegetables; stir in dressing. Cover and refrigerate until serving. **Yield:** 8 servings.

TO COOK FRESH CORN. Plunge husked ears into a large kettle of boiling water. Don't salt during cooking, since salt can harden kernels. Boil until tender, about 8 to 10 minutes, less for just-picked corn.

Exchanges: 1 Starch

Nutritional Information

Serving Size: 1/2 cup
Calories: 64
Sodium: 93 mg
Cholesterol: 0

Carbohydrate: 15 gm
Protein: 2 gm
Fat: 1 gm

Fresh Broccoli Salad

Marilyn Fields, Groveland, California

*When time is short and you want something delicious,
this recipe fills the bill. It has great crunch, and the dressing is
quick to make. This colorful salad goes fast at potlucks.*

2 pounds fresh broccoli, cut into
  bite-size pieces
1 package (12 ounces) fresh
  mushrooms, sliced
2 small red onions, thinly sliced
  into rings
1 can (2-1/4 ounces) sliced ripe
  olives, drained
1-1/2 cups low-fat Italian salad
  dressing
  1/3 cup shredded Parmesan
  cheese

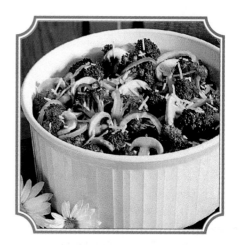

Combine all ingredients in a large bowl;
toss to mix well. Cover and chill for at
least 2 hours. **Yield:** 12 servings.

Exchanges: 2 Vegetable, 1/2 Fat

Nutritional Information

Serving Size: 1 cup
Calories: 66
Sodium: 182 mg
Cholesterol: 3 mg

Carbohydrate: 9 gm
Protein: 5 gm
Fat: 2 gm

Tomato Strip Salad

Mary Jo Amos, Noel, Missouri

Between attending college, working as an emergency room clerk and serving on church council, I'm often cooking meals just for myself. So this single-serving salad really comes in handy.

1 tomato, peeled, seeded and cut into strips
1/4 cup fresh *or* frozen peas, parboiled
2 tablespoons fresh green chili strips
1/2 teaspoon lemon juice
1/2 teaspoon minced fresh cilantro *or* parsley
Lettuce leaves

In a bowl, toss tomato strips, peas, chili strips, lemon juice and cilantro or parsley. Cover and chill. Serve on a bed of lettuce. **Yield:** 1 serving.

TOMATO TIP. For best flavor, purchase tomatoes ripened on the vine in an area near you. Those shipped long distances are picked green and are less flavorful as they ripen in stores.

Exchanges: 1 Vegetable, 1/2 Starch
Nutritional Information

Serving Size: 1 recipe
Calories: 61
Sodium: 48 mg
Cholesterol: 0

Carbohydrate: 12 gm
Protein: 3 gm
Fat: 1 gm

Eggplant Salad

Elizabeth Roper, Norfolk, Virginia

*This recipe has been passed down through the family,
starting with my grandmother, who learned it from her neighbor.
It's a delightful way to prepare eggplant.*

**1 medium eggplant (about 1-1/4
  pounds)**
**4 medium tomatoes, cubed
  (3-1/2 to 4 cups)**
3 hard-cooked eggs, cubed
1 large onion, chopped
**1/2 cup low-fat French salad
  dressing**
1/2 teaspoon pepper

Cut eggplant in half lengthwise. Place
with cut side down in a greased 9-in.
square baking dish. Bake at 350° for 30-
40 minutes or until tender. Cool, peel and
cut the eggplant into 1/2-in. cubes; place
in a large salad bowl. Add tomatoes, eggs
and onion. Add dressing and pepper; toss.

Cover and chill 1 hour before serving.
Yield: 10 servings.

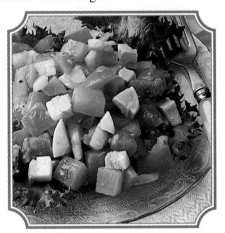

Exchanges: 2 Vegetable, 1/2 Fat
Nutritional Information

Serving Size: 1/10 recipe
Calories: 76
Sodium: 268 mg
Cholesterol: 62 mg

Carbohydrate: 10 gm
Protein: 3 gm
Fat: 3 gm

Tomato Vinaigrette

Donna Aho, Fargo, North Dakota

My mother-in-law gave me this recipe years ago, and I've used it often ever since. It's a nice change of pace from your basic lettuce and tomato salad.

12 thick tomato slices
1/2 cup olive oil
2 to 3 tablespoons red wine vinegar
1 garlic clove, minced
1 teaspoon snipped fresh oregano
1/2 teaspoon salt
1/4 teaspoon pepper
1/4 teaspoon dry mustard
6 large lettuce leaves
Minced green onions
Minced fresh parsley

Arrange tomato slices in an 8-in. square dish; set aside. In a small bowl, whisk together oil, vinegar, garlic, oregano, salt, pepper and mustard. Pour over tomatoes. Cover and chill for 1-2 hours. To serve, place each lettuce leaf on an individual plate and top with two tomato slices. Drizzle with dressing. Sprinkle with onions and parsley. **Yield:** 6 servings.

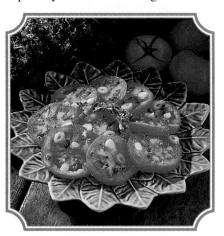

Exchanges: 3 Fat, 1 Vegetable

Nutritional Information

Serving Size: 2 tomato slices
Calories: 174
Sodium: 197 mg
Cholesterol: 0

Carbohydrate: 3 gm
Protein: 1 gm
Fat: 18 gm

Green Salad with Dill Dressing

Lucy Meyring, Walden, Colorado

The creamy, easy-to-prepare dressing in this recipe turns an ordinary green salad into a spectacular treat. I like to make this pretty side dish year-round, but especially at the holidays.

1 head Boston lettuce, torn
1/2 bunch romaine, torn
4 green onions, sliced
3 radishes, sliced
1 large green pepper, cut into strips
1 large tomato, diced
1 carrot, shredded
1 small cucumber, sliced
DILL DRESSING:
2 tablespoons red wine vinegar
1 teaspoon Dijon mustard
2 tablespoons light sour cream
1/4 cup vegetable oil
3 tablespoons olive oil
2 teaspoons dill weed

In a large bowl, combine the first eight ingredients. Refrigerate. For dressing, whisk the vinegar and mustard in a small bowl. Whisk in remaining ingredients. Refrigerate for at least 30 minutes. Stir well before serving with the salad. **Yield:** 8 servings (about 3/4 cup dressing).

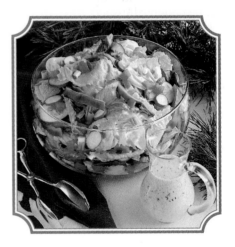

Exchanges: 1-1/2 Fat, 1 Vegetable

Nutritional Information

Serving Size: 1/8 salad recipe with 1 tablespoon dressing
Calories: 101
Sodium: 20 mg

Cholesterol: 0
Carbohydrate: 7 gm
Protein: 3 gm
Fat: 9 gm

Kansas Cucumber Salad

Karen Ann Bland, Gove, Kansas

Cucumbers are my favorite garden vegetable, so I use this recipe often. A friend shared it with me quite a few years ago. I've heard this dish keeps well in the refrigerator, but it goes so fast around our house I've never found out for myself!

1 cup low-fat mayonnaise
1/4 cup sugar
4 teaspoons vinegar
1/2 teaspoon dill weed
4 medium cucumbers, peeled and thinly sliced
3 green onions, chopped

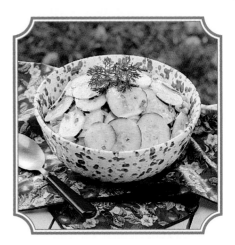

In a large bowl, combine mayonnaise, sugar, vinegar and dill; mix well. Add cucumbers and onions; toss. Cover and chill for at least 1 hour. **Yield:** 8 servings.

Exchanges: 2 Vegetable, 1-1/2 Fat

Nutritional Information

Serving Size: 2/3 cup
Calories: 126
Sodium: 197 mg
Cholesterol: 6 mg

Carbohydrate: 14 gm
Protein: 1 gm
Fat: 8 gm

Golden Glow Salad

Thelma Waggoner, Hopkinsville, Kentucky

My sister and I loved this salad when we were growing up because we thought it tasted like a dessert. I always make this salad for picnics. It provides a fruit and a vegetable, and bright color as well.

1 package (.3 ounce) sugar-free
  orange-flavored gelatin
1 cup boiling water
1 can (8 ounces) crushed pineapple
  in natural juices
1 tablespoon lemon juice
Cold water
  3/4 cup finely shredded carrots

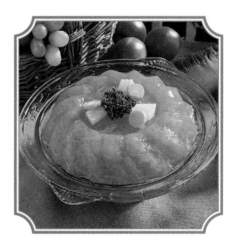

In a bowl, dissolve gelatin in boiling water. Drain pineapple, reserving juice. Add lemon juice and enough cold water to pineapple juice to make 1 cup. Stir into gelatin. Chill until slightly set. Stir in pineapple and carrots. Pour into a 4-cup mold coated with nonstick cooking spray; cover and chill until firm. Unmold. **Yield:** 6 servings.

Exchanges: 1/2 Fruit

Nutritional Information

Serving Size: 1/6 recipe
Calories: 35
Sodium: 42 mg
Cholesterol: 0

Carbohydrate: 8 gm
Protein: trace
Fat: 0

Strawberry Salad

Ruth Barton, Millsap, Texas

*Even though it's low-fat, this fresh and fruity salad is
always a hit at church dinners and family reunions.
My sister shared this recipe with me many years ago.*

2 cups unsweetened frozen
    strawberries
2 ripe bananas
Artificial sweetener equivalent to 2
    tablespoons sugar
    1 package (.6 ounce) sugar-free
        strawberry-flavored gelatin
    2 cups boiling water
    1 can (8 ounces) crushed
        pineapple in natural juices,
        undrained
    1 carton (8 ounces) plain low-fat
        yogurt

In a bowl, mash strawberries, bananas
and sweetener; set aside. In another
bowl, dissolve gelatin in boiling water.
Stir in strawberry mixture and pineapple.
Pour half into an 8-in. square dish. Chill
until firm. Combine yogurt and remaining gelatin mixture; spoon over chilled
strawberry mixture. Chill until firm.
Yield: 8 servings.

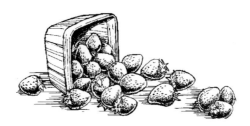

Exchanges: 1 Fruit, 1/4 Skim Milk
Nutritional Information

Serving Size: 1/8 recipe
Calories: 86
Sodium: 76 mg
Cholesterol: 2 mg

Carbohydrate: 18 gm
Protein: 3 gm
Fat: 1 gm

Fruit Salad Supreme

Lois Rutherford, St. Augustine, Florida

For a delightful fruit salad that's a snap to prepare, give this recipe a try. The sweet combination, topped with onion and a tangy dressing, is one family and friends ask for often. It's also one of my favorites to serve.

2 cups watercress, stems
    removed
8 fresh pineapple rings, halved
2 oranges, peeled and sliced
    crosswise
1-1/2 cups cantaloupe chunks
1/4 cup sliced green onions *or* 1
    small sweet onion, chopped
LIME DRESSING:
1/4 cup vegetable oil
2 tablespoons lime juice
1 tablespoon sugar
1/4 teaspoon hot pepper sauce
1 tablespoon light sour cream

On individual plates, arrange watercress, pineapple and oranges. Top with cantaloupe and onions. In a small bowl, whisk oil, lime juice, sugar and hot pepper sauce until sugar is dissolved. Stir in sour cream. Serve with salads. **Yield:** 4 servings.

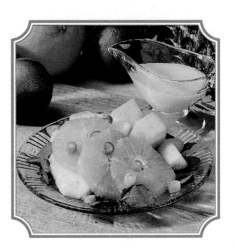

Exchanges: 3 Fat, 1-1/2 Fruit

Nutritional Information

Serving Size: 1/4 salad recipe
with 2 tablespoons dressing
Calories: 216
Sodium: 15 mg

Cholesterol: 0
Carbohydrate: 27 gm
Protein: 2 gm
Fat: 15 gm

Orange Blossom Salad

Dorothy Anderson, Ottawa, Kansas

Packed with fruits and vegetables, this lively salad is nice year-round—both for everyday dinners and special-occasion meals. Best of all, it can be assembled in no time, so it's perfect for busy cooks.

3 oranges, peeled and sectioned
2 cups cauliflowerets
1/4 cup chopped green pepper
2 cups torn fresh spinach
DRESSING:
  1 can (12 ounces) evaporated
  skim milk
  1 can (6 ounces) frozen orange
  juice concentrate, thawed

In a large salad bowl, combine orange segments, cauliflower, green pepper and spinach. Place dressing ingredients in a jar with a tight-fitting lid; shake until well mixed. Serve dressing on side. Refrigerate leftover dressing. **Yield:** 6 servings (2 cups dressing).

"A-PEEL-ING" TIP. Before discarding unused orange peels, grate the rind—avoiding the white zest—and freeze in small amounts for future baking and cooking.

Exchanges: 1 Vegetable, 1/2 Fruit
Nutritional Information

Serving Size: 1/6 salad recipe with 1 tablespoon dressing
Calories: 62
Sodium: 47 mg

Cholesterol: trace
Carbohydrate: 13 gm
Protein: 3 gm
Fat: trace

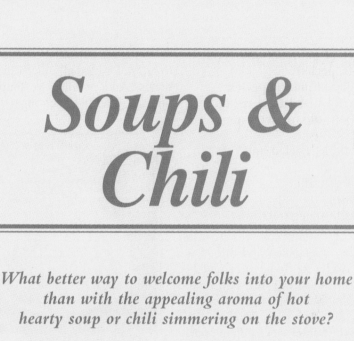

Soups & Chili

What better way to welcome folks into your home than with the appealing aroma of hot hearty soup or chili simmering on the stove?

Dilled Chicken Soup

Estelle Keefer, Allegany, New York

Everyone who tries this soup says it's the best they've ever tasted.
I like it because I can put it all together and let it simmer
while I get chores done around the house.

1 chicken (4 pounds), quartered
3 carrots, peeled
1 small sweet potato, peeled
4 celery ribs with leaves, cut up
1 small parsnip, peeled and
  sliced
1 large onion, peeled and
  quartered
Few sprigs fresh dill
Pepper to taste
8 ounces thin egg noodles,
  cooked and drained

Place chicken, vegetables and dill in a large kettle. Add water to cover, about 2-1/2 qts. Cover and bring to a boil over high heat. Skim foam. Add pepper; cover and simmer for 2 hours. Remove the chicken and vegetables; set aside to cool. Pour the broth through a strainer; skim fat. Slice carrots and dice chicken; return to broth. Discard all other vegetables and bones. Add noodles to soup and heat through. **Yield:** 10 servings.

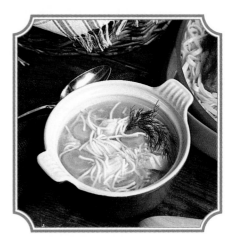

Exchanges: 3 Very Lean Meat, 1 Starch, 1/2 Vegetable

Nutritional Information

Serving Size: 1/10 recipe
Calories: 207
Sodium: 62 mg
Cholesterol: 73 mg

Carbohydrate: 19 gm
Protein: 22 gm
Fat: 4 gm

Chunky Chili

Verna Hofer, Mitchell, South Dakota

I love to cook and bake, especially when our children and grandchildren are here. After spending time outdoors, this chili warms up the coldest winter evening!

1-1/2 pounds lean chuck *or* round steak, cut into bite-size pieces
1 tablespoon cooking oil
2 garlic cloves, minced
2 green peppers, chopped
1 large onion, chopped
1 to 3 tablespoons chili powder
2 teaspoons ground cumin
1 teaspoon dried oregano
1 can (28 ounces) low-sodium tomatoes with liquid, chopped
1 can (15 to 16 ounces) kidney beans, rinsed and drained

In a large heavy saucepan, cook meat in oil until lightly browned. Add next seven ingredients; bring to a boil. Reduce heat and simmer, covered, for 2-1/2 to 3 hours or until meat is tender. Stir in beans during the last 30 minutes of cooking. **Yield:** 7 servings.

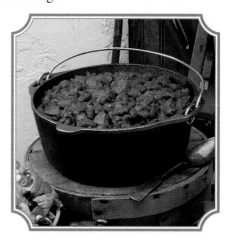

Exchanges: 3 Lean Meat, 1 Vegetable, 1 Starch

Nutritional Information

Serving Size: 1 cup
Calories: 253
Sodium: 321 mg
Cholesterol: 57 mg

Carbohydrate: 22 gm
Protein: 27 gm
Fat: 7 gm

Steak Soup

Mary Dice, Chemainus, British Columbia

One of the nice things about this thick soup is you can make it in an afternoon without too much fuss.

2 tablespoons margarine
2 tablespoons cooking oil
1-1/2 pounds lean round steak, cut
    into 1/2-inch cubes
1/4 cup chopped onion
3 tablespoons all-purpose flour
1 tablespoon paprika
1/4 teaspoon pepper
4 cups low-sodium beef broth
2 cups water
1 bay leaf
4 sprigs fresh parsley, chopped
2 sprigs celery leaves, chopped
1/2 teaspoon dried marjoram
1-1/2 cups cubed peeled potatoes
1-1/2 cups sliced carrots
1-1/2 cups chopped celery
1 can (6 ounces) low-sodium
    tomato paste

In a Dutch oven, melt margarine over medium heat; add oil. Brown beef and onion. Combine flour, paprika and pepper; sprinkle over beef and mix well. Stir in stock and water. Add bay leaf, parsley, celery leaves and marjoram; bring to a boil. Reduce heat; cover and simmer about 1 hour or until meat is tender. Add potatoes, carrots and celery. Cover and simmer for 30-45 minutes or until vegetables are tender and soup begins to thicken. Stir in tomato paste; simmer, uncovered, for 15 minutes. Remove bay leaf before serving. **Yield:** 6 servings.

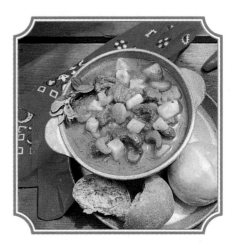

Exchanges: 3 Meat, 1 Starch, 1 Vegetable

Nutritional Information

Serving Size: 1/6 recipe
Calories: 325
Sodium: 185 mg
Cholesterol: 67 mg

Carbohydrate: 20 gm
Protein: 29 gm
Fat: 14 gm

Vegetable Bean Soup

Laura Letobar, Livonia, Michigan

On cold winter days, my family likes to sit down to steaming bowlfuls of this fabulous soup. It's packed with hearty vegetables and beans and has a unique robust flavor.

2 cups chopped onion
1 cup chopped carrots
1 cup chopped celery
6 cups water
3 low-sodium beef bouillon cubes
1 can (28 ounces) low-sodium tomatoes with liquid, cut up
1 can (15 ounces) black beans, rinsed and drained
1 cup quick-cooking barley
1 teaspoon garlic powder
3/4 teaspoon pepper
1 package (10 ounces) frozen chopped spinach, thawed

In a large saucepan or Dutch oven coated with nonstick cooking spray, saute onion, carrots and celery over medium heat until onion is soft, about 8 minutes. Stir in water, bouillon, tomatoes, beans, barley, garlic powder and pepper; bring to a boil. Reduce heat; cover and simmer for 10 minutes. Add spinach; cover and simmer for 10-15 minutes or until the vegetables are tender. **Yield:** 14 servings.

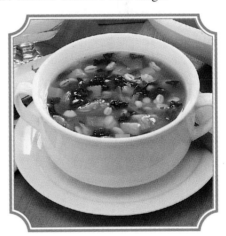

Exchanges: 1 Starch, 1 Vegetable

Nutritional Information

Serving Size: 1/14 recipe
Calories: 113
Sodium: 254 mg
Cholesterol: 0

Carbohydrate: 23 gm
Protein: 6 gm
Fat: 1 gm

Chicken Barley Soup

Diana Costello, Marion, Kansas

No question—this is my favorite soup. It's so filling that I serve it as a hearty main dish, and I have given the recipe to many of our friends and relatives. It tastes too good to keep to yourself!

1 broiler-fryer chicken (3 pounds), cut up
2 quarts water
1-1/2 cups diced carrots
1 cup diced celery
1/2 cup barley
1/2 cup chopped onion
1 bay leaf
1/2 teaspoon poultry seasoning
1/2 teaspoon pepper
1/2 teaspoon dried sage

In a large kettle, cook chicken in water until tender. Cool broth and skim off fat. Bone the chicken and cut into bite-size pieces; return to kettle along with remaining ingredients. Cover and simmer for at least 1 hour or until vegetables and barley are tender. Remove bay leaf before serving. **Yield:** 5 servings.

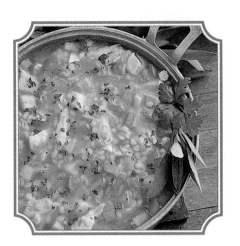

Exchanges: 2-1/2 Lean Meat, 1 Starch, 1 Vegetable
Nutritional Information
Serving Size: 1 cup
Calories: 259
Sodium: 127 mg
Cholesterol: 89 mg

Carbohydrate: 22 gm
Protein: 31 gm
Fat: 5 gm

Beef Lentil Soup

Constance Turnbull, Arlington, Massachusetts

You can prepare this soup as the main course for a hearty lunch or dinner. But—on cold winter evenings here in New England—I often pour a mugful and enjoy sipping it in front of our fireplace as well.

1 pound lean ground beef
1 quart water
1 can (48 ounces) tomato juice
1 cup dry lentils, rinsed
2 cups chopped cabbage
1 cup sliced carrots
1 cup sliced celery
1 cup chopped onion
1/2 cup diced green pepper
1/2 teaspoon pepper
1/2 teaspoon dried thyme
1 bay leaf
1 package (10 ounces) frozen chopped spinach, thawed

In a large kettle, brown ground beef. Drain. Add water, tomato juice, lentils, cabbage, carrots, celery, onion, green pepper, pepper, thyme and bay leaf. Bring to a boil. Reduce heat and simmer, un-covered, for 1 to 1-1/2 hours or until the lentils and vegetables are tender. Add spinach and heat through. Remove bay leaf before serving. **Yield:** 6 servings.

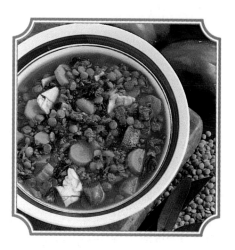

Exchanges: 2 Meat, 2 Vegetable, 1-1/2 Starch
Nutritional Information

Serving Size: 1/6 recipe
Calories: 317
Sodium: 128 mg
Cholesterol: 45 mg

Carbohydrate: 38 gm
Protein: 28 gm
Fat: 7 gm

Herbed Chicken Soup

Myrna Huebert, Tofield, Alberta

I love cooking from scratch and turning a recipe into my own personal "creation". This soup is one I developed gradually over the years...after some experimenting.

1 broiler-fryer chicken (3-1/2 pounds), cut up
2-1/2 quarts water
4 medium carrots, cut into 1/2-inch pieces
1 medium onion, chopped
1/2 cup chopped celery
5 low-sodium chicken bouillon cubes
2 tablespoons dried parsley flakes
1 tablespoon dried thyme
1 teaspoon *each* dried sage and poultry seasoning
1/2 teaspoon pepper
1 large bay leaf
1 package (12 ounces) frozen noodles *or* 2 cups cooked noodles

In a 4-qt. soup kettle, place all ingredients except noodles. Cover and bring to a boil; skim fat. Reduce heat; cover and and simmer for 1-1/2 hours or until chicken is tender. Remove chicken; allow to cool. Debone and cut into chunks. Skim fat from broth; bring to a boil. Return chicken to kettle. Add frozen noodles and cook for 20 minutes or until tender, or add cooked noodles and heat through. Remove bay leaf. **Yield:** 16 servings.

Exchanges: 1 Lean Meat, 1/2 Starch
Nutritional Information

Serving Size: 1 cup
Calories: 91
Sodium: 181 mg
Cholesterol: 31 mg

Carbohydrate: 8 gm
Protein: 11 gm
Fat: 2 gm

Quick Chili

Jean Ward, Montgomery, Texas

*Who says great-tasting chili has to simmer all day long?
I've been making this easy—yet hearty—version for some
34 years, much to the delight of family and friends.*

**1 pound lean ground beef
1 can (10-3/4 ounces) low-fat,
low-sodium condensed tomato
soup, undiluted
1 can (15 ounces) chili beans in
gravy, undrained
2 to 3 teaspoons chili powder
1/2 cup water, optional**

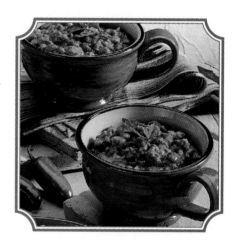

In a saucepan, brown the ground beef;
drain. Add soup, beans and chili powder.
Reduce heat. Cover and simmer for 20
minutes. Add water if a thinner soup is desired. **Yield:** 4 servings.

Exchanges: 3 Meat, 1-1/2 Starch
Nutritional Information
Serving Size: 1/4 recipe
Calories: 344
Sodium: 341 mg
Cholesterol: 108 mg

Carbohydrate: 24 gm
Protein: 31 gm
Fat: 5 gm

Mushroom/Onion Soup

Nancy Kuczynski, Holmen, Wisconsin

*Even folks who don't like mushrooms have a hard time resisting this soup!
I've found it's a great first course when I have friends over for dinner.*

2 cups (8 ounces) fresh mushrooms
3 tablespoons margarine
2 medium onions, chopped
2 tablespoons all-purpose flour
5 cups low-sodium chicken broth
Dash pepper
1/3 cup uncooked long grain rice
1 bay leaf
2 tablespoons chopped fresh
parsley

Trim mushroom stems level with the caps; finely chop stems and thinly slice caps. In a large saucepan, melt margarine; add mushrooms and onions. Cook and stir over low heat for 5 minutes. Blend in flour; add broth and pepper. Cook, stirring constantly, until mixture boils. Reduce heat. Add rice and bay leaf; cover and simmer for 15-20 minutes or until the rice is tender. Discard bay leaf. Sprinkle with parsley. **Yield:** 4 servings.

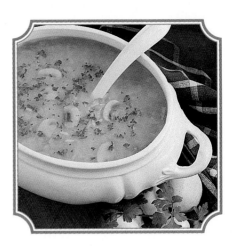

Exchanges: 1 Vegetable, 1 Fat, 1/2 Starch
Nutritional Information

Serving Size: 1-1/4 cups
Calories: 118
Sodium: 26 mg
Cholesterol: 1 mg

Carbohydrate: 10 gm
Protein: 8 gm
Fat: 5 gm

Hoosier Chili

Jeanne Boberg, Muncie, Indiana

*This chili is a little sweeter than other recipes I've tasted,
but I like it that way. It reminds me of the chili my mom used to make.*

2 pounds extra-lean ground beef
2 cups chopped onion
3/4 cup chopped celery
1/2 cup chopped green pepper
3 garlic cloves, minced
1/4 teaspoon pepper
1 tablespoon brown sugar
3 tablespoons chili powder
**2 cans (16 ounces *each*) sodium-
free stewed tomatoes**
**1 can (46 ounces) sodium-free
tomato juice**
1 cup water
1 low-sodium beef bouillon cube
1/2 cup uncooked elbow macaroni
**1 can (15 to 16 ounces) kidney
beans, rinsed and drained**

In a large Dutch oven or soup kettle, brown beef until no longer pink. Add onion, celery, green pepper and garlic. Continue cooking until vegetables are tender. Add all remaining ingredients except last two; bring to a boil. Reduce heat; cover and simmer for 1-1/2 hours, adding macaroni for last half hour of cooking time. Stir in the beans and heat through. **Yield:** 12 servings.

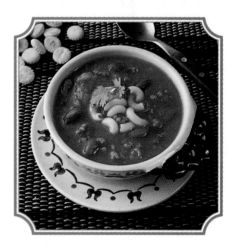

Exchanges: 2 Meat, 1-1/2 Vegetable, 1 Starch
Nutritional Information

Serving Size: 1 cup
Calories: 255
Sodium: 68 mg
Cholesterol: 45 mg

Carbohydrate: 23 gm
Protein: 18 gm
Fat: 13 gm

Turkey Soup

Carol Brethauer, Denver, Colorado

I especially enjoy preparing this soup around the holidays after a big turkey dinner. But my family enjoys it so much that I find myself making it year-round.

1 turkey carcass
3 quarts water
2 cans (10-1/2 ounces *each*)
  low-sodium chicken broth
1/2 cup uncooked long grain rice
1 medium onion, finely chopped
4 celery ribs, finely chopped
2 carrots, grated
1 bay leaf
Dash poultry seasoning
Pepper, onion powder and garlic
  powder to taste

Place turkey carcass, water and broth in a large soup kettle. Simmer over low heat for 4-5 hours. Remove carcass from stock. Remove any meat and dice; skim fat. Return to stock along with rice, onion, celery, carrots, bay leaf and poultry seasoning. Add remaining seasonings. Simmer over medium-low heat until the rice is cooked. **Yield:** 8 servings (3 quarts).

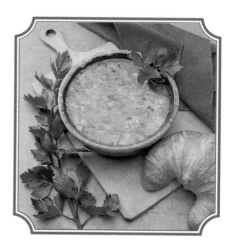

Exchanges: 1 Lean Meat, 1/2 Starch
Nutritional Information

Serving Size: 1-1/2 cups
(turkey meat estimated at 1 oz.)
Calories: 95
Sodium: 54 mg

Cholesterol: 21 mg
Carbohydrate: 9 gm
Protein: 10 gm
Fat: 2 gm

Zesty Steak Chili

Michelle Smith, Running Springs, California

*A pot of hearty chili is always welcome when weather starts turning cooler.
This full-flavored, medium–hot chili tastes even better the second day.*

**4 pounds round steak, cut into
    1-inch cubes**
4 garlic cloves, minced
1/4 cup cooking oil
3 cups chopped onion
2-3/4 cups water, *divided*
2 cups sliced celery
**3 cans (14-1/2 ounces *each*)
    diced tomatoes, undrained**
**2 cans (15 ounces *each*) no-salt
    tomato sauce**
1 jar (16 ounces) salsa
3 tablespoons chili powder
2 teaspoons ground cumin
2 teaspoons dried oregano
1 teaspoon pepper
1/4 cup all-purpose flour
1/4 cup yellow cornmeal

In a Dutch oven over medium-high heat, saute steak and garlic in oil until browned. Add onion; cook and stir for 5 minutes. Stir in 2 cups water and next eight ingredients; bring to a boil. Reduce heat; cover and simmer 2 hours or until tender. Combine flour, cornmeal and remaining water; stir until smooth. Bring chili to a boil. Add flour mixture; cook and stir 2 minutes or until thickened. If desired, garnish with low-fat cheese, light sour cream, onions and olives. **Yield:** 20 servings.

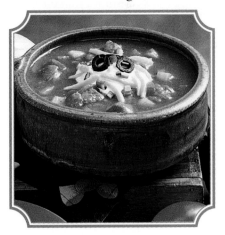

Exchanges: 2 Meat, 2 Vegetable
Nutritional Information

Serving Size: 1 cup
Calories: 187
Sodium: 155 mg
Cholesterol: 44 mg

Carbohydrate: 13 gm
Protein: 19 gm
Fat: 7 gm
(Calculated without garnishes)

Hearty Navy Bean Soup

Mildred Lewis, Temple, Texas

Beans were a commodity you did not survive without in the '30's.
This excellent bean soup is a real family favorite of ours and I make it often.

**3 cups (1-1/2 pounds) dry navy
    beans
1 can (16 ounces) tomatoes
    with liquid, cut up
1 large onion, chopped
1 cup diced fully cooked lean ham
2 cups low-sodium chicken broth
2-1/2 cups water
Pepper to taste
Chopped fresh parsley**

Rinse and sort beans. Cover with cold water and soak overnight. Drain beans and place in a large soup kettle or Dutch oven. Add tomatoes with liquid, onion, ham, broth, water and pepper. Bring to a boil. Reduce heat; cover and simmer until beans are tender, about 1-1/2 hours. Add more water if necessary. (For a thicker soup, beans may be pureed in a food processor or blender and then returned to the kettle and heated through.) Garnish with parsley. **Yield:** 10 servings.

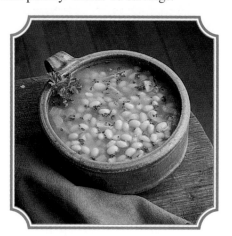

Exchanges: 2-1/2 Starch, 1 Lean Meat, 1 Vegetable

Nutritional Information

Serving Size: 1/10 recipe
Calories: 265
Sodium: 373 mg
Cholesterol: 10 mg

Carbohydrate: 41 gm
Protein: 19 gm
Fat: 3 gm

Barley Borscht

Blanche Babinski, Minto, North Dakota

This is one of my favorite soups. It makes good use of the many vegetables that are harvested each fall here in North Dakota.

2 pounds beef bones
1 medium onion, chopped
1 bay leaf
1 teaspoon salt
10 whole peppercorns
6 cups water
1 medium rutabaga (about 1 pound), diced
3 cups diced fresh beets (about 1-1/2 pounds)
2 cups chopped celery
1 small head cabbage (about 1 pound), shredded
2-1/2 cups diced carrots (about 1 pound)
2-1/2 cups diced peeled potatoes (about 1 pound)

3/4 cup pearl barley
1 can (14-1/2 ounces) low-sodium tomatoes with liquid, cut up
1/4 cup vinegar

In a Dutch oven, combine beef bones, onion, bay leaf, salt, peppercorns and water. Bring to a boil; reduce heat. Cover and simmer for 2 hours. Strain broth; discard bones, onion and seasonings. Skim fat and return broth to the kettle. Add rutabaga, beets, celery, cabbage, carrots, potatoes and barley. Return to a boil; reduce heat. Cover and simmer 50 minutes or until vegetables are almost tender and barley is cooked. Stir in tomatoes with liquid and vinegar; heat through. **Yield:** 16 servings.

Exchanges: 1 Starch, 1 Vegetable
Nutritional Information
Serving Size: 1 cup
Calories: 110
Sodium: 227 mg
Cholesterol: 0
Carbohydrate: 26 gm
Protein: 3 gm
Fat: 1 gm

Creamy Carrot Soup

Bertha McClung, Summersville, West Virginia

This blended soup is loaded with vegetables, so it's delicious as well as good for you. Plus, its special golden color adds a special touch to your table.

3 cups thinly sliced carrots
1 cup chopped onion
2/3 cup chopped celery
1-1/2 cups diced peeled potatoes
1 garlic clove, minced
1/2 teaspoon sugar
2 teaspoons cooking oil
4 cups low-sodium chicken broth
Dash ground nutmeg
Pepper to taste

In a Dutch oven or soup kettle over medium-low heat, saute carrots, onion, celery, potatoes, garlic and sugar in oil for 5 minutes. Add broth, nutmeg and pepper; bring to a boil. Reduce heat; cover and simmer for 30-40 minutes or until vegetables are tender. Remove from the heat and cool to room temperature. Puree in batches in a blender or food processor. Return to the kettle and heat through. **Yield:** 4 servings.

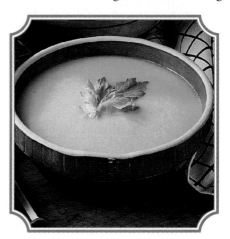

Exchanges: 2 Vegetable, 1 Starch, 1/2 Fat
Nutritional Information

Serving Size: 1-1/2 cups
Calories: 136
Sodium: 116 mg
Cholesterol: 0

Carbohydrate: 23 gm
Protein: 5 gm
Fat: 3 gm

Gazpacho

Chris Brooks, Prescott, Arizona

"Simple as can be" best describes this hearty cold soup. You just chop and combine the ingredients, then chill for a few hours. It tastes great with crunchy croutons or breadsticks.

1 can (46 ounces) vegetable juice
1 can (10-1/2 ounces) condensed
   beef consomme, undiluted
2 cups chopped cucumber
2 cups chopped tomatoes
1 cup chopped green pepper
1/2 cup chopped onion
1/2 cup chopped celery

1/3 cup red wine vinegar
2 tablespoons fresh lemon juice
2 garlic cloves, minced
3 to 4 drops hot pepper sauce

In a large bowl, combine all ingredients; mix well. Cover and chill for 2-3 hours before serving. Serve cold. **Yield:** 12 servings.

> **JUICY TIP.** When tomatoes are in season, why not blend your own juice in a food processor? Use it in this recipe or as a beverage.

Exchanges: 2 Vegetable

Nutritional Information

Serving Size: 1 cup
Calories: 52
Sodium: 470 mg
Cholesterol: 0

Carbohydrate: 11 gm
Protein: 3 gm
Fat: trace

Garden Harvest Chili

Judy Sloter, Charles City, Iowa

I started making my chili back when we lived near a huge farmers' market that sold all sorts of vegetables. My husband likes this better than traditional chili.

2 tablespoons cooking oil
2 garlic cloves, minced
1 medium green pepper, chopped
1 medium sweet red pepper, chopped
1-1/2 cups sliced fresh mushrooms
1/2 cup chopped onion
1 can (28 ounces) tomatoes with liquid, cut up
1 can (15 ounces) low-sodium tomato sauce
2 tablespoons chili powder
2 teaspoons sugar
1 teaspoon ground cumin
1 can (15 to 16 ounces) kidney beans, rinsed and drained
2 cups sliced zucchini
1 package (10 ounces) frozen sweet corn, thawed
Shredded low-fat cheddar cheese, optional

In a skillet, heat oil over medium-high. Saute garlic, peppers, mushrooms and onion until tender. Add tomatoes with liquid, tomato sauce, chili powder, sugar and cumin; heat to boiling. Reduce heat to low; add beans, zucchini and corn. Simmer, uncovered, about 10 minutes or until zucchini is tender. Spoon into bowls; sprinkle with cheese if desired. **Yield:** 6 servings.

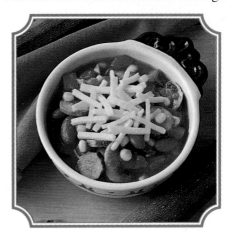

Exchanges: 2 Starch, 2 Vegetable, 1 Fat
Nutritional Information
Serving Size: 1-3/4 cups
Calories: 252
Sodium: 675 mg
Cholesterol: 0

Carbohydrate: 44 gm
Protein: 10 gm
Fat: 7 gm
(Calculated without cheese garnish)

Peasant Soup

Bertha McClung, Summersville, West Virginia

One taste and you'll agree this soup is anything but meager. The hearty vegetable broth really satisfies, and it's inexpensive to make as well.

1 pound dry great northern beans
3 carrots, sliced
3 celery ribs, sliced
2 medium onions, chopped
2 garlic cloves, minced
2 bay leaves
1 can (14-1/2 ounces) tomatoes
  with liquid, cut up
1 teaspoon dried basil
1/2 teaspoon pepper
2 tablespoons olive oil

Place the beans in a Dutch oven and cover with water; bring to a boil. Boil for 2 minutes. Remove from the heat; cover and let stand for 1 hour. Drain and rinse beans; return to Dutch oven. Add 6 cups water, carrots, celery, onions, garlic, bay leaves, tomatoes, basil and pepper; bring to a boil. Reduce heat; cover and simmer for 1-1/2 hours or until the beans are tender. Discard the bay leaves. Add oil and heat through. **Yield:** 12 servings.

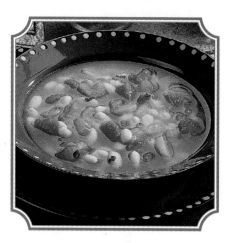

Exchanges: 1 Vegetable, 1 Starch, 1/2 Lean Meat, 1/2 Fat

Nutritional Information

Serving Size: 1 cup
Calories: 140
Sodium: 73 mg
Cholesterol: 0 mg

Carbohydrate: 22 gm
Protein: 8 gm
Fat: 3 gm

White Chili

Lana Rutledge, Shepherdsville, Kentucky

This is one of my favorite recipes because the chili simmers all day in a slow cooker. When your hungry clan calls for dinner, you can ladle up steaming bowlfuls in a hurry.

2 medium onions, chopped
4 garlic cloves, minced
2 quarts water
3 pounds chicken breasts, skin removed
1 pound dry navy beans
2 cans (4 ounces *each*) chopped green chilies
1 tablespoon ground cumin
2 teaspoons dried oregano
1/2 to 1 teaspoon cayenne pepper
1/2 teaspoon ground cloves
2 low-sodium chicken bouillon cubes
Dried chives and crushed red pepper flakes, optional

Place onions and garlic in the bottom of a slow cooker. Add the next nine ingredients; do not stir. Cook on high for 8-10 hours. Uncover and stir (meat should fall off the bones). Remove bones. Stir to break up the meat. Spoon into bowls; sprinkle with chives and red pepper flakes if desired. **Yield:** 12 servings.

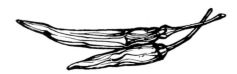

Exchanges: 3 Lean Meat, 2 Starch

Nutritional Information

Serving Size: 1 cup
Calories: 294
Sodium: 239 mg
Cholesterol: 73 mg

Carbohydrate: 28 gm
Protein: 37 gm
Fat: 4 gm

Peoria Chili

Norma Erne, Albuquerque, New Mexico

*I remember coming home from school on cold days to a
warm kitchen and smelling Mom's chili simmering on the stove.
Why not create your own mmm-memories with this recipe?*

2 pounds ground beef
1 medium onion, chopped
1 can (28 ounces) tomatoes with
  liquid, cut up
1 can (46 ounces) tomato juice
1 to 2 tablespoons chili powder
1 tablespoon sugar
Pepper to taste
  2 cans (15 to 16 ounces *each*)
    kidney beans, rinsed and drained
Low-fat shredded cheddar cheese,
  optional

In a large kettle or Dutch oven, brown
beef and onion. Drain off fat; add all remaining ingredients except beans and
cheese. Cover and simmer 2-3 hours. Stir
in beans and heat through. Garnish with
cheese if desired. **Yield:** 10 servings.

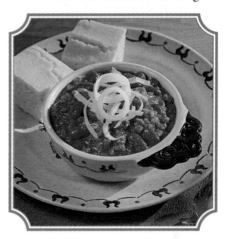

Exchanges: 3 Lean Meat, 1-1/2 Starch, 1 Vegetable
Nutritional Information
Serving Size: 1/10 recipe
Calories: 288
Sodium: 826 mg
Cholesterol: 64 mg

Carbohydrate: 28 gm
Protein: 26 gm
Fat: 9 gm
(Calculated without cheese garnish)

Rosemary Split Pea Soup

Diane Hixon, Niceville, Florida

The addition of rosemary and meatballs make this a new and interesting version of typical split pea soup. I like to serve it as a meal in itself.

3 celery ribs, finely chopped
1 cup finely chopped onion
1 garlic clove, minced
1 tablespoon fresh rosemary, minced *or* 1 teaspoon dried rosemary, crushed
3 tablespoons margarine
6 cups low-sodium chicken broth
1-1/4 cups dry split peas, rinsed
MEATBALLS:
1/2 pound ground turkey breast
1-1/2 teaspoons fresh rosemary, minced *or* 1/2 teaspoon dried rosemary, crushed
1/4 teaspoon pepper

In a large kettle or Dutch oven, saute celery, onion, garlic and rosemary in margarine until tender. Add broth and peas; bring to a boil. Reduce heat; cover and simmer for 1-1/2 hours or until peas are soft. Remove from the heat and allow to cool. For meatballs, combine turkey, rosemary and pepper. Shape into 1/2-in. balls. In a skillet, brown meatballs until no pink remains, about 5-10 minutes. Ladle half of the cooled soup into a blender or food processor; puree. Return soup to the kettle along with the meatballs and heat through. **Yield:** 5 servings.

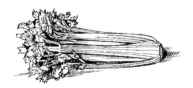

Exchanges: 3 Lean Meat, 2 Starch, 1 Vegetable

Nutritional Information

Serving Size: 1/5 recipe
Calories: 354
Sodium: 213 mg
Cholesterol: 24 mg

Carbohydrate: 38 gm
Protein: 30 gm
Fat: 10 gm

Beef Minestrone

Ann Lape, Richmondville, New York

This recipe pleasantly proves that decreasing fat intake doesn't mean saying farewell to ground beef's full-bodied flavor. This soup is sure to be a hit in your home.

1 pound ground round
1 cup chopped onion
6 cups water
1 cup cubed peeled potatoes
1 cup chopped tomatoes
1 cup shredded cabbage
1 cup chopped carrots
1/2 cup chopped celery
1/4 cup uncooked long grain rice
1/2 teaspoon dried basil
1/2 teaspoon dried thyme

1 bay leaf
1/4 teaspoon pepper
5 teaspoons grated Parmesan cheese

In a Dutch oven, cook meat and onion until meat is browned and onion is tender; drain. Add next 11 ingredients; bring to a boil. Reduce heat; cover and simmer for 1 hour. Discard bay leaf. Sprinkle each serving with 1/2 teaspoon of Parmesan. **Yield:** 10 servings.

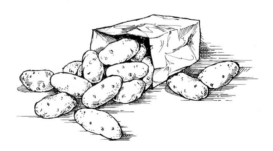

Exchanges: 1 Meat, 1 Vegetable, 1/2 Starch
Nutritional Information

Serving Size: 1 cup
Calories: 141
Sodium: 58 mg
Cholesterol: 31 mg

Carbohydrate: 10 gm
Protein: 11 gm
Fat: 7 gm

Chicken Chili with Black Beans

Jeanette Urbom, Overland Park, Kansas

Because it looks different than traditional chili, my family was a little hesitant to try this dish at first. But thanks to full, hearty flavor, it's become a real favorite.

3 whole boneless skinless chicken breasts (about 1-3/4 pounds), cubed
2 medium sweet red peppers, chopped
1 large onion, chopped
4 garlic cloves, minced
3 tablespoons olive oil
1 can (4 ounces) chopped green chilies
2 tablespoons chili powder
2 teaspoons ground cumin
1 teaspoon ground coriander
2 cans (15 ounces *each*) black beans, rinsed and drained
1 can (28 ounces) Italian plum tomatoes with liquid, chopped
1 cup chicken broth

In a Dutch oven, saute chicken, red peppers, onion and garlic in oil for 5 minutes or until chicken is no longer pink. Add green chilies, chili powder, cumin and coriander; cook for 3 minutes. Stir in beans, tomatoes and broth; bring to a boil. Reduce heat and simmer, uncovered, for 15 minutes, stirring often. **Yield:** 10 servings (3 quarts).

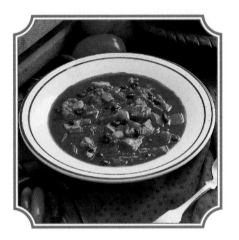

Exchanges: 1 Meat, 1 Vegetable, 1/2 Starch
Nutritional Information
Serving Size: 1-1/4 cups
Calories: 149
Sodium: 172 mg
Cholesterol: 33 mg

Carbohydrate: 12 gm
Protein: 16 gm
Fat: 4 gm

Barley Broccoli Soup

Gloria Porter, Grandin, North Dakota

This original recipe of mine was a winner in a barley soup contest. Barley makes it hearty and nutritious—and it's a good way to use broccoli or asparagus from your garden.

3 cups water
3 low-sodium beef bouillon cubes
1/2 cup medium pearl barley
2 cups fresh *or* frozen chopped broccoli *or* asparagus, cooked and drained
4 cups skim milk
5 slices American cheese
1/4 teaspoon ground nutmeg
1/4 teaspoon pepper

In a saucepan, bring water, bouillon and barley to a boil. Reduce heat; cover and simmer for 50-60 minutes or until barley is tender and nearly all liquid is absorbed. Stir often but do not drain. Add broccoli or asparagus. Stir in milk, cheese, nutmeg and pepper. Heat through, stirring often, until soup is hot and cheese is melted. **Yield:** 8 servings.

SOUPER SIMPLE MEALS. If you're cooking for one or two, there's no need to cut soup recipes in half. Simply freeze leftovers in serving-size portions for quick-and-easy meals later.

Exchanges: 1 Meat, 1/2 Skim Milk, 1/2 Starch
Nutritional Information

Serving Size: 1/8 recipe
Calories: 145
Sodium: 285 mg
Cholesterol: 15 mg

Carbohydrate: 17 gm
Protein: 9 gm
Fat: 5 gm

Swedish Potato Dumpling Soup

Margaret Peterson, Genoa, Nebraska

*Family and friends gather around our table throughout
the year to enjoy good company and great food.
This hearty soup is part of our traditional Christmas meal.*

1 broiler-fryer chicken (3-1/2 pounds), cut up
6-1/2 cups water
2 celery ribs, quartered
1 medium carrot, quartered
1 small onion, peeled
4 whole peppercorns
2 whole cloves
2 whole allspice
2 low-sodium chicken bouillon cubes
1 package (10 ounces) frozen green beans
1 package (12 ounces) frozen noodles

DUMPLINGS:
2 medium potatoes, cooked and mashed (without added milk or butter)
Egg substitute equivalent to 1 egg
2 tablespoons half-and-half cream
1 teaspoon sugar
1/2 cup all-purpose flour

In a 5-qt. soup kettle, combine the first nine ingredients. Cover and bring to a boil. Reduce heat; simmer for 3 hours. Remove chicken; allow to cool. Strain broth, discarding vegetables and seasonings; skim fat. Add enough water to make 8 cups; return to kettle. Debone chicken and cut into chunks; add to kettle with beans and noodles. Bring to a boil; cook for 20 minutes. For dumplings, mix potatoes, egg substitute, cream and sugar in a medium bowl. Gradually add flour to make a stiff batter (it should form a peak when spoon is lifted). Drop by teaspoons into boiling soup. Cover and simmer for 3 minutes. **Yield:** 12 servings.

Exchanges: 2 Lean Meat, 1 Starch
Nutritional Information
Serving Size: 1 cup
Calories: 192
Sodium: 62 mg
Cholesterol: 52 mg
Carbohydrate: 15 gm
Protein: 19 gm
Fat: 6 gm

Buffalo Chili Con Carne

Donna Smith, Victor, New York

This classic recipe of the American frontier is so meaty you can almost eat it with a fork. The zippy combination of vegetables, beans and seasonings is a perfect complement to the buffalo.

1 pound cubed *or* coarsely ground buffalo meat
2 tablespoons cooking oil
1 to 2 cups diced onion
1 to 2 cups diced green pepper
2 cans (16 ounces *each*) diced tomatoes with liquid
1-1/2 to 2 cups tomato juice
1 can (15 to 16 ounces) kidney beans, rinsed and drained
1 can (15 ounces) pinto beans, rinsed and drained
1 can (4 ounces) chopped green chilies
2 teaspoons chili powder
1/2 teaspoon pepper

In a large kettle or Dutch oven, brown meat in oil; drain. Add onion and green pepper; saute for 5 minutes. Stir in remaining ingredients and bring to a boil. Reduce heat; cover and simmer 1-1/2 to 2 hours or until the meat is tender. **Yield:** 6 servings.

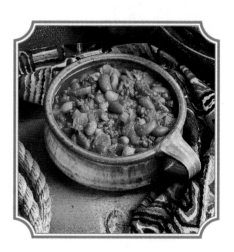

Exchanges: 2 Lean Meat, 2 Starch, 1 Vegetable

Nutritional Information

Serving Size: 1 cup
Calories: 271
Sodium: 574 mg
Cholesterol: 27 mg

Carbohydrate: 39 gm
Protein: 23 gm
Fat: 3 gm

Five-Bean Soup

Lynne Dodd, Mentor, Ohio

One of my family's favorite soups, this tasty recipe was one I discovered years ago. Served with a salad and bread or rolls, it makes a savory supper.

**5 packages (1 pound *each*)
  dry beans: lima, great northern,
  kidney, pinto and split peas
  (enough for four batches
  of soup)
3 low-sodium beef bouillon cubes
3 tablespoons dried chives
1 teaspoon dried savory
1/2 teaspoon ground cumin
1/2 teaspoon pepper
1 bay leaf
2-1/2 quarts water
1 can (14-1/2 ounces) stewed
  tomatoes**

Combine beans; divide into four equal batches, about 3-3/4 cups each. *To make one batch of soup:* Wash one batch of beans. Place in a large kettle; add enough water to cover. Bring to a boil; cook for 3-4 minutes. Remove from heat; cover and let stand 1 hour. Tie spices in a cheesecloth bag. Drain and rinse beans. Return to kettle; add bouillon, spices and water. Bring to boil. Reduce heat; cover and simmer 1-1/2 hours or until beans are tender, stirring occasionally. Remove spices. Add tomatoes and heat through. **Yield:** one batch makes 14 servings.

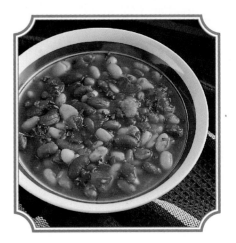

Exchanges: 2 Starch, 1 Vegetable, 1/2 Meat
Nutritional Information
Serving Size: 1 cup
Calories: 191
Sodium: 293 mg
Cholesterol: 0

Carbohydrate: 35 gm
Protein: 13 gm
Fat: 1 gm

'Forgotten' Minestrone

Marsha Ransom, South Haven, Michigan

This soup gets its name because the broth simmers for hours, allowing me to work on my free-lance writing. But after one taste, you and your family will agree this full-flavored soup is truly unforgettable!

1 pound lean beef stew meat
6 cups water
1 can (28 ounces) tomatoes with liquid, cut up
1 low-sodium beef bouillon cube
1 medium onion, chopped
2 tablespoons minced dried parsley
1-1/2 teaspoons ground thyme
1/2 teaspoon pepper
1 medium zucchini, thinly sliced
2 cups finely chopped cabbage
1 can (16 ounces) garbanzo beans, rinsed and drained
1 cup uncooked small elbow *or* shell macaroni

In a slow cooker, combine beef, water, tomatoes, bouillon, onion, parsley, thyme and pepper. Cover and cook on low for 7-9 hours or until meat is tender. Add zucchini, cabbage, beans and macaroni; cook on high, covered, 30-45 minutes more or until the macaroni and vegetables are tender. **Yield:** 8 servings.

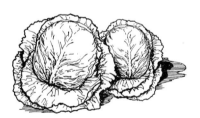

Exchanges: 2 Vegetable, 1-1/2 Starch, 1 Meat
Nutritional Information
Serving Size: 1/8 recipe
Calories: 246
Sodium: 342 mg
Cholesterol: 33 mg

Carbohydrate: 30 gm
Protein: 19 gm
Fat: 6 gm

Vegetarian Chili

Barb Gumieny, Wauwatosa, Wisconsin

This recipe teams rice with hearty kidney and pinto beans and a variety of colorful vegetables for a deliciously healthy meatless meal. Your family is sure to love it.

1 medium green pepper, chopped
1 medium onion, chopped
3 garlic cloves, minced
1 tablespoon cooking oil
2 cans (14-1/2 ounces *each*) Mexican-style stewed tomatoes
1 can (15 to 16 ounces) kidney beans, rinsed and drained
1 can (15 ounces) pinto beans, rinsed and drained
1 can (11 ounces) whole kernel corn, drained
2-1/2 cups water
1 cup uncooked long grain rice
1 to 2 tablespoons chili powder
1-1/2 teaspoons ground cumin

In a Dutch oven, saute green pepper, onion and garlic in oil until tender. Stir in all remaining ingredients; bring to a boil. Reduce heat; cover and simmer for 25-30 minutes or until rice is cooked, stirring occasionally. If thinner chili is desired, add additional water. **Yield:** 11 servings.

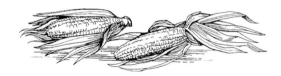

Exchanges: 2 Starch, 2 Vegetable
Nutritional Information

Serving Size: 1 cup
Calories: 191
Sodium: 616 mg
Cholesterol: 0

Carbohydrate: 38 gm
Protein: 7 gm
Fat: 2 gm

Cucumber Potato Soup

Robert Breno, Strongsville, Ohio

Served hot or cold, this soup never fails to delight the taste buds. It's simple to make, has a nice dill flavor and is a great way to use a few potatoes and a garden cucumber.

4 medium potatoes, peeled and diced
1 teaspoon salt
2 cups water
1 medium cucumber, peeled, seeded and diced
1/4 teaspoon white pepper
1-1/2 cups skim milk
1 green onion, sliced
1 teaspoon dill weed *or* 1 tablespoon chopped fresh dill

In a large saucepan, combine potatoes, salt and water; cook until potatoes are very soft. Place sieve over a large bowl. Pour potatoes and liquid into sieve and force potatoes through. Return to saucepan. Stir in cucumber, pepper, milk and onion. Simmer gently for about 5 minutes or until cucumber is tender. Add dill. Serve hot or cold. **Yield:** 4 servings.

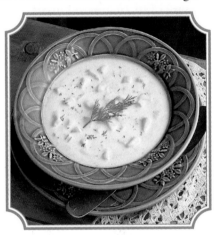

Exchanges: 1 Starch, 1 Vegetable, 1/2 Skim Milk

Nutritional Information

Serving Size: 1/4 recipe
Calories: 131
Sodium: 631 mg
Cholesterol: 2 mg

Carbohydrate: 27 gm
Protein: 6 gm
Fat: trace

Easy Low-Fat Chili

Janet Moore, Ogdensburg, New York

This recipe proves you don't have to prepare a five-course meal in order to enjoy a satisfying supper. This zesty chili will really hit the spot throughout the year when you serve it with a simple salad and bread.

1 medium onion, chopped
1/4 cup chopped green pepper
4 cups water, *divided*
1 can (15 to 16 ounces) great northern beans, rinsed and drained
1 can (15 ounces) navy beans, rinsed and drained
1 can (6 ounces) salt-free tomato paste
1 can (14-1/2 ounces) low-sodium diced tomatoes with liquid
2 to 4 teaspoons chili powder
1/2 teaspoon pepper

In a large saucepan, cook the onion and green pepper in 1/2 cup water until tender. Add beans, tomato paste and tomatoes. Stir in chili powder, pepper and remaining water; bring to a boil. Reduce heat; cover and simmer for 20 minutes. **Yield:** 7 servings.

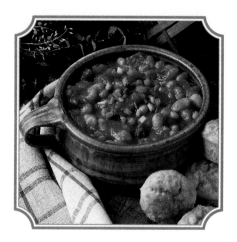

Exchanges: 2 Starch, 1-1/2 Vegetable

Nutritional Information

Serving Size: 1 cup
Calories: 198
Sodium: 295 mg
Cholesterol: 0

Carbohydrate: 38 gm
Protein: 11 gm
Fat: 1 gm

Garden Vegetable Soup

Dorothy Miller, Royersford, Pennsylvania

*During the Depression, our garden was the source for most of our food.
I can remember picking fresh vegetables and then enjoying the
mouth-watering aroma as this soup simmered for hours.*

1 small head cabbage (about 1
  pound), chopped
3 medium green peppers, chopped
2 medium sweet red peppers,
  chopped
5 medium onions, chopped
3 celery ribs, chopped
6 medium tomatoes, peeled,
  seeded and chopped *or* 1 can
  (28 ounces) tomatoes with
  liquid, cut up
4 cups low-sodium chicken broth
1 bay leaf
1 tablespoon chopped fresh
  parsley *or* 1 teaspoon dried
  parsley flakes
1/4 teaspoon dried thyme
1/4 teaspoon garlic powder
Pepper to taste

Combine all ingredients in a large kettle
or Dutch oven; bring to a boil. Reduce
heat. Cover and simmer for 2-1/2 hours or
until vegetables are tender, stirring occasionally. Remove the bay leaf before serving. **Yield:** 10 servings.

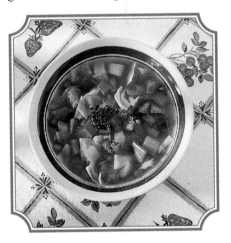

Exchanges: 1 Vegetable, 1/2 Starch
Nutritional Information

Serving Size: 1/10 recipe
Calories: 64
Sodium: 39 mg
Cholesterol: 0

Carbohydrate: 15 gm
Protein: 4 gm
Fat: 1 gm

Granny's Spicy Soup

Rose Rose, Akron, Ohio

My mother makes the best soups around and has become known as "The Soup Lady". When my kids ask me to make Granny's soup, I'm happy to oblige. I look forward to this soup's robust flavor as much as they do.

1 broiler-fryer chicken (4 pounds), cut up
2 quarts water
5 celery ribs with leaves, diced
2 medium carrots, diced
1 large onion, diced
1-1/2 teaspoons pickling spices
4 low-sodium chicken bouillon cubes
1/4 teaspoon pepper
1 cup uncooked noodles

Place chicken and water in a large soup kettle. Cover and bring to a boil; skim fat. Reduce heat; cover and simmer for 2 hours or until chicken falls off bone. Strain broth; return to kettle. Allow chicken to cool; debone and cut into chunks. Skim fat from broth. Return chicken to broth along with celery, carrots and onion. Place pickling spices in a tea ball or cheesecloth bag; add to soup. Bring to a boil. Reduce heat; cover and simmer for 1 hour. Remove spices; add bouillon, pepper and noodles. Cook for 10-15 minutes or until noodles are tender. **Yield:** 12 servings. **Editor's Note:** The soup gets its name from the pickling spices, not from being hot.

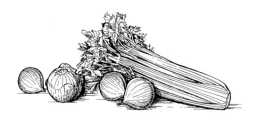

Exchanges: 1 Lean Meat, 1 Vegetable, 1/2 Starch

Nutritional Information

Serving Size: 1 cup
Calories: 114
Sodium: 74 mg
Cholesterol: 32 mg

Carbohydrate: 9 gm
Protein: 14 gm
Fat: 3 gm

Tomato Dill Bisque

Susan Breckbill, Lincoln University, Pennsylvania

*My family really enjoys this soup when we make it from our garden tomatoes.
When those tomatoes are plentiful, I make a big batch and freeze it.
Then we can enjoy it even after the garden is gone for the season.*

2 medium onions, chopped
1 garlic clove, minced
2 tablespoons margarine
2 pounds tomatoes, peeled and
　chopped
1/2 cup water
1 low-sodium chicken bouillon cube
1 teaspoon sugar
1 teaspoon dill weed
1/2 teaspoon salt
1/4 teaspoon pepper

In a large saucepan, saute onions and garlic in margarine until tender. Add tomatoes, water, bouillon, sugar and seasonings. Cover and simmer 10 minutes or until tomatoes are tender. Remove from heat; cool. Puree in a blender or food processor.

Return to saucepan. Cook and stir over low heat until heated through. Serve warm. **Yield:** 5 servings.

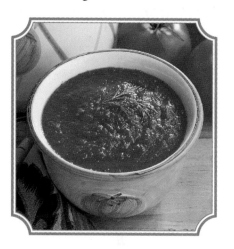

Exchanges: 2 Vegetable, 1 Fat

Nutritional Information

Serving Size: 1 cup
Calories: 108
Sodium: 285 mg
Cholesterol: 0

Carbohydrate: 14 gm
Protein: 3 gm
Fat: 5 gm

Chunky Chicken Soup

Kathy Both, Rocky Mountain House, Alberta

Here's a satisfying soup that you'll find yourself serving year-round. Every spoonful is loaded with the fantastic flavor of chicken, celery, carrots and peas. No matter how much I make, it seems to disappear quickly.

3 boneless skinless chicken thighs, cut into 1-inch pieces
1 cup sliced celery
1/2 cup chopped onion
2 tablespoons cooking oil
6 cups low-sodium chicken broth
1-1/2 cups sliced carrots
1 teaspoon dried thyme
1/4 teaspoon pepper
1/2 cup uncooked macaroni
1-1/2 cups frozen peas

In a 3-qt. saucepan, cook chicken, celery and onion in oil until chicken juices run clear. Add broth, carrots, thyme and pepper; bring to a boil. Reduce heat; cover and simmer for 45 minutes or until vegetables are tender. Stir in macaroni and peas. Cover and simmer for 15 minutes or until macaroni is tender. **Yield:** 8 servings.

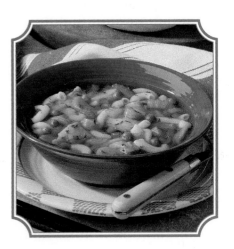

Exchanges: 1 Starch, 1 Meat

Nutritional Information

Serving Size: 1 cup
Calories: 140
Sodium: 109 mg
Cholesterol: 18 mg

Carbohydrate: 13 gm
Protein: 10 gm
Fat: 6 gm

Creamy Vegetable Soup

Rita Zagrzebski, Eagle River, Wisconsin

*I like to watch my diet but hate to sacrifice flavor in order to reduce fat.
That's why this recipe is such a delight. No one will ever guess
this delicious creamy soup is actually good for you!*

3 cans (14-1/2 ounces *each*) low-
  sodium chicken broth
4 carrots, chopped
2 medium unpeeled potatoes,
  chopped
2 medium onions, chopped
1/2 cup uncooked brown rice
8 cups coarsely chopped fresh
  broccoli
8 cups coarsely chopped fresh
  cauliflower
4 cups skim milk
1/4 teaspoon pepper

In a large kettle, combine broth, carrots, potatoes, onions and rice; cover and bring to a boil. Reduce heat; simmer for 20 minutes. Add broccoli and cauliflower; simmer for 20 minutes or until the vegetables are tender. Cool slightly. Puree half of the mixture in a blender or food processor; return to kettle. Add milk and pepper; mix well. Heat through (do not boil). **Yield:** 18 servings.

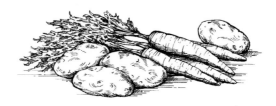

Exchanges: 1 Vegetable, 1/2 Starch, 1/2 Skim Milk
Nutritional Information
Serving Size: 1 cup
Calories: 105
Sodium: 83 mg
Cholesterol: 1 mg

Carbohydrate: 17 gm
Protein: 6 gm
Fat: 1 gm

Harvest Chicken Rice Soup

Diane Winningham, Uniontown, Missouri

*Because the produce in this soup is pureed, you can easily get
children to eat their vegetables…without them knowing it!
Kids of all ages will surely savor this classic soup.*

2 celery ribs with leaves
2 medium carrots
1 pound white potatoes, peeled
1 pound sweet potatoes, peeled
3 quarts water
2 pounds broiler-fryer chicken
 pieces, skin removed
2 large onions, halved
3 low-sodium chicken bouillon
 cubes
3 cups cooked rice (prepared
 without added salt)
Pepper to taste

Cut vegetables into 2-in. pieces; place in a 5-qt. Dutch oven. Add water, chicken, onions and bouillon. Bring to a boil; skim fat. Reduce heat; cover and simmer for 2 hours. Remove from the heat. Remove chicken and allow both broth and chicken to cool to lukewarm; skim fat. Puree the vegetables and broth in a blender; strain. Debone chicken and cut into chunks. Return chicken and broth to Dutch oven. Stir in rice. Cook over medium heat until bubbly, stirring occasionally. Season with pepper. **Yield:** 20 servings.

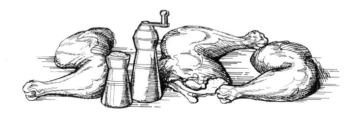

Exchanges: 1-1/2 Lean Meat, 1 Starch, 1 Vegetable
Nutritional Information

Serving Size: 1 cup
Calories: 174
Sodium: 57 mg
Cholesterol: 41 mg

Carbohydrate: 19 gm
Protein: 15 gm
Fat: 4 gm

Southwestern Chicken Soup

Joe Greenough, Bedford, Texas

This is the first recipe I've ever devised in its entirety and I'm proud to say family and friends seem pleased with the results. I like this soup a little spicy, but it can easily be modified to suit anyone's tastes.

2/3 cup low-sodium beef broth
1 can (12 ounces) no-salt tomato paste
1 can (15 to 16 ounces) kidney beans, rinsed and drained
1 can (11 ounces) Mexican-style corn, drained
1-1/2 cups diced cooked chicken
3 green onions, sliced
2 to 3 tablespoons chili powder
1 can (4 ounces) chopped green chilies
1-2/3 cups water

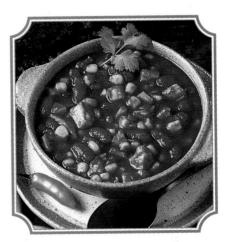

In a large saucepan, combine beef broth and tomato paste. Add remaining ingredients. Cover and simmer for 20 minutes. **Yield:** 6 servings.

Exchanges: 1-1/2 Starch, 1-1/2 Lean Meat, 1 Vegetable

Nutritional Information

Serving Size: 1/6 recipe
Calories: 224
Sodium: 631 mg
Cholesterol: 21 mg

Carbohydrate: 32 gm
Protein: 20 gm
Fat: 3 gm

Chicken Chili

Janne Rowe, Wichita, Kansas

This unique and delicious chicken chili is a much-requested meal around our house. I think you'll find it's a nice change of pace from the typical beef version.

3 cups chopped onion
1-1/2 cups chopped green pepper
4 garlic cloves, minced
2 tablespoons cooking oil
1-1/2 pounds boneless skinless chicken breasts, cut into 1/2-inch cubes
2 to 4 tablespoons chili powder
1 tablespoon ground cumin
2 teaspoons ground coriander
1/2 teaspoon cayenne pepper
2 cans (14-1/2 ounces *each*) low-sodium diced tomatoes with liquid
2 cans (10-1/2 ounces *each*) condensed low-sodium chicken broth
2 cups water
1 can (6 ounces) tomato paste
1 bay leaf
2 cans (15 ounces *each*) garbanzo beans, rinsed and drained

In a 5-qt. Dutch oven, cook onion, green pepper and garlic in oil over medium-high heat for 10 minutes or until onion is tender. Add chicken; cook and stir constantly for 4 minutes or until browned. Add the next nine ingredients; bring to a boil. Reduce heat; cover and simmer, stirring occasionally, for 40 minutes. Add beans; cook, uncovered, for 20 minutes, stirring occasionally. Remove bay leaf. **Yield:** 14 servings.

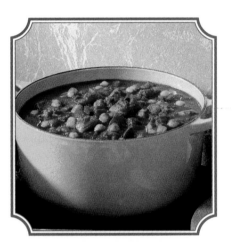

Exchanges: 2 Lean Meat, 1 Starch, 1 Vegetable
Nutritional Information
Serving Size: 1 cup
Calories: 222
Sodium: 230 mg
Cholesterol: 49 mg

Carbohydrate: 26 gm
Protein: 18 gm
Fat: 6 gm

Tomato Barley Soup

Jeannine Fournier, Concord, Vermont

I serve this attractive soup as a mouth-watering meal after a day of skiing and sledding. Everyone who samples it comments on the robust tomato taste.

4-1/2   pounds broiler-fryer chicken pieces, skin removed
4   quarts water
6   large carrots, sliced
5   medium onions, chopped
2   cups sliced celery
1   tablespoon minced fresh parsley
2   teaspoons dried rosemary, crushed
1-1/2   teaspoons dried thyme
1-1/2   teaspoons dried savory
1/2   teaspoon pepper
1   cup uncooked brown rice
1/2   cup pearl barley
1   bottle (32 ounces) low-sodium tomato juice
1   can (28 ounces) crushed tomatoes

In an 8-qt. soup kettle, combine the first 10 ingredients. Cover and bring to a boil. Reduce heat; simmer for 2 hours. Remove chicken; allow to cool. Skim fat from broth. Debone chicken and cut into chunks; return to kettle. Add remaining ingredients; bring to a boil. Reduce heat; cover and simmer for 1 hour or until barley and rice are tender. **Yield:** 28 servings.

Exchanges: 1 Lean Meat, 1 Vegetable, 1/2 Starch
Nutritional Information
Serving Size: 1 cup
Calories: 105
Sodium: 110 mg
Cholesterol: 21 mg
Carbohydrate: 14 gm
Protein: 9 gm
Fat: 2 gm

Tex-Mex Chicken Soup

MayDell Spiess, Industry, Texas

We keep busy here on our ranch, so I'm always looking for dishes that can be prepared in a hurry but are still filling and tasty. This soup is a real winner!

1/2 cup chopped onion
2 garlic cloves, minced
1 tablespoon cooking oil
4 cups low-sodium chicken broth
3 cups cubed cooked chicken
3 medium zucchini, sliced
1 can (14-1/2 ounces) low-sodium tomatoes with liquid, cut up
1 can (11 ounces) low-sodium whole kernel corn, drained
1 can (8 ounces) low-sodium tomato sauce
1/2 cup salsa
2 teaspoons ground cumin
3/4 teaspoon pepper
1/2 teaspoon dried oregano
Shredded low-fat cheddar cheese, optional

In a 4-qt. soup kettle, saute onion and garlic in oil until tender. Add the next 10 ingredients; bring to a boil. Reduce heat; cover and simmer for 30 minutes. If desired, garnish individual servings with cheese. **Yield:** 12 servings.

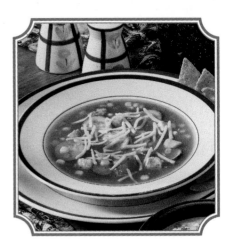

Exchanges: 1 Vegetable, 1/2 Starch, 1/2 Fat

Nutritional Information

Serving Size: 1 cup
Calories: 91
Sodium: 109 mg
Cholesterol: 21 mg

Carbohydrate: 10 gm
Protein: 8 gm
Fat: 3 gm
(Calculated without cheese garnish)

Mom's Tomato Vegetable Soup

Sandra Davis, Brownsville, Tennessee

I developed this soup from a recipe my mom made often. Its robust down-home taste brings back wonderful memories of growing up on our farm.

1 broiler-fryer chicken (3 pounds), cut up
8 cups water
1 celery rib, halved
1 medium onion, halved
3 medium potatoes, peeled and cut into 1/2-inch cubes
2 cups low-sodium tomato juice
1 can (16 ounces) mixed vegetables, drained
1 can (15-1/2 ounces) black-eyed peas, rinsed and drained
1 can (14-1/2 ounces) low-sodium stewed tomatoes
1/2 cup chopped onion
1 teaspoon pepper
1/2 pound lean ground beef
1 can (15 ounces) cream-style corn

In an 8-qt. soup kettle, place chicken, water, celery and onion. Cover and bring to a boil; skim fat. Reduce heat; cover and simmer for 1-1/2 hours or until chicken falls off the bones. Strain broth and skim fat; return broth to kettle. Add the next seven ingredients. Debone chicken and cut into chunks; return to kettle. Bring to a boil. Meanwhile, in a medium skillet, brown beef; drain and add to soup. Reduce heat; cover and simmer for 1 hour. Stir in corn; cook, uncovered, for 30 minutes, stirring occasionally. **Yield:** 18 servings.

HANDY HELPFUL HINT. Always thaw ground beef in the refrigerator—never at room temperature. Brown the beef until pink no longer remains and drain thoroughly.

Exchanges: 1 Meat, 1 Vegetable, 1/2 Starch

Nutritional Information

Serving Size: 1 cup
Calories: 155
Sodium: 69 mg
Cholesterol: 31 mg

Carbohydrate: 15 gm
Protein: 14 gm
Fat: 4 gm

Veggie Chicken Chili

Lois Leininger, Grants Pass, Oregon

Because this chili freezes well, I like to keep some on hand for dinner on busy days or for last-minute entertaining.

2 tablespoons cooking oil
4 cups chopped fresh broccoli
1 large leek *or* 4 green onions (white part only), chopped
1 medium red onion, chopped
1 medium sweet red pepper, chopped
1 medium green pepper, chopped
1 large carrot, chopped
2/3 cup chopped celery
3 garlic cloves, minced
5 cups low-sodium chicken broth, *divided*
4 cups cubed cooked chicken
2 cans (15 to 16 ounces *each*) kidney beans, rinsed and drained
1 can (28 ounces) low-sodium diced tomatoes with liquid
1 can (4 ounces) chopped green chilies
1/4 cup packed brown sugar
2 tablespoons *each* ground cumin, ground coriander and dried oregano
2 tablespoons Worcestershire sauce
1/2 cup cornstarch
3 tablespoons chili powder

In an 8-qt. soup kettle, heat oil. Add next eight ingredients; mix well. Cover and cook over medium-low heat for 15 minutes or until vegetables are slightly softened. Add 4 cups broth, chicken, beans, tomatoes, chilies, brown sugar, cumin, coriander, oregano and Worcestershire sauce. Bring to a boil; reduce heat. Cover and simmer for 1 hour, stirring occasionally. Combine cornstarch, chili powder and remaining broth; stir into chili. Cook and stir until thickened. **Yield:** 20 servings.

Exchanges: 1 Starch, 1 Lean Meat, 1 Vegetable

Nutritional Information

Serving Size: 1 cup
Calories: 138
Sodium: 121 mg
Cholesterol: 17 mg

Carbohydrate: 19 gm
Protein: 11 gm
Fat: 3 gm

Beef

Some mighty meaty eating is right at your fingertips with these hearty main meals. So round up your hungry clan and dig in!

Oriental Beef and Cauliflower Stew

Deborah Cole, Wolf Creek, Oregon

Next to hamburger, round steak probably is the most frequent dinner "guest" at our place! I'm always experimenting with recipes...this one's easy and good.

2 tablespoons cooking oil
1-1/2 pounds lean round steak, cut into 1-inch cubes
3 cups beef broth
1 small head cauliflower, separated into florets
1 green pepper, cut into chunks
1/4 cup light soy sauce
1 garlic clove, minced
1-1/2 teaspoons grated fresh gingerroot, optional
2 to 3 tablespoons cornstarch
1/2 teaspoon sugar
1/4 cup water
1 cup sliced green onions
Hot cooked rice, optional

In a skillet, heat oil over medium-high. Brown meat on all sides. Add broth; cover and simmer until beef is tender, about 1 hour. Add cauliflower, green pepper, soy sauce, garlic and gingerroot if de-sired. Cover and simmer until the vegetables are tender, about 5-7 minutes. Combine cornstarch, sugar and water. Stir into meat mixture. Bring to a boil, stirring constantly; cook 2 minutes or until thickened. Stir in green onions. Serve over rice if desired. **Yield:** 6 servings.

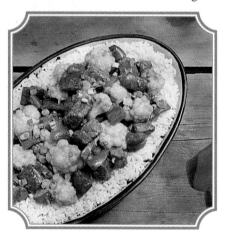

Exchanges: 2-1/2 Lean Meat, 1 Vegetable
Nutritional Information

Serving Size: 1/6 recipe
Calories: 165
Sodium: 771 mg
Cholesterol: 82 mg

Carbohydrate: 8 gm
Protein: 23 gm
Fat: 4 gm
(Calculated without rice)

Mushroom Beef Skillet

Vicki Raatz, Waterloo, Wisconsin

I like to serve this impressive-looking skillet supper for special dinners with family and friends. I think you'll agree it's a wonderfully flavorful "slimmed down" version of traditional beef Stroganoff.

1 pound flank steak
2 cups low-sodium beef broth
1 cup chopped onion
1 pound fresh mushrooms,
  sliced
1/4 cup cold water
2 tablespoons all-purpose flour
2 tablespoons cornstarch
1/2 cup plain fat-free yogurt
1 teaspoon paprika
1 teaspoon prepared mustard
1/2 teaspoon garlic powder

Broil steak 6 in. from the heat until rare, about 5 minutes on each side. Cut diagonally into thin strips; set aside and keep warm. In a large skillet, bring broth to a boil. Add onion and mushrooms; cover and simmer until tender, about 5 minutes. In a small bowl, mix cold water, flour and cornstarch until smooth. Whisk into broth; cook and stir over low heat until thickened and bubbly. Remove from heat. In a bowl, combine yogurt, paprika, mustard and garlic powder; add to broth and stir until smooth. Add the beef; cook over low heat, stirring constantly, until heated through, about 5 minutes. **Yield:** 6 servings.

Exchanges: 2 Meat, 1 Vegetable, 1/2 Starch
Nutritional Information

Serving Size: 1/6 recipe
Calories: 239
Sodium: 103 mg
Cholesterol: 47 mg

Carbohydrate: 13 gm
Protein: 21 gm
Fat: 11 gm

Steak Lo Mein

Jo Groth, Plainfield, Iowa

My family likes chow mein...this is a little like that but not quite as exotic. Stir-fry dishes are a favorite at our house.

1 pound round steak, trimmed
1 teaspoon low-sodium beef
 bouillon granules
3/4 cup water
1/4 cup soy sauce
2 tablespoons cornstarch
2 tablespoons cooking oil
1 garlic clove, minced
2 cups shredded cabbage
1 cup diagonally sliced carrots,
 partially cooked
1 medium onion, sliced into rings
1/2 cup sliced fresh mushrooms
1/2 cup diagonally sliced celery
1/3 cup sliced green onions
15 fresh snow peas, trimmed
1 can (8 ounces) sliced water
 chestnuts, drained
4 ounces thin spaghetti,
 cooked and drained

Freeze steak just until firm; slice diagonally across grain into 1/4-in. strips. Combine bouillon, water, soy sauce and cornstarch; set aside. In a wok or large skillet, heat oil on medium-high. Add meat and garlic; stir-fry until the meat is no longer pink, about 5 minutes. Remove meat to a platter. Add cabbage, carrots, onion, mushrooms, celery and green onions; stir-fry for about 3 minutes. Add peas and water chestnuts; stir-fry 2 minutes. Add meat. Stir bouillon mixture and pour into skillet; cook and stir until thickened. Gently toss in spaghetti and heat through for 1 minute. **Yield:** 6 servings.

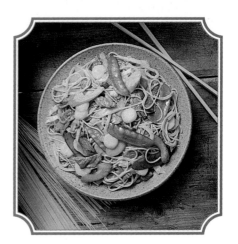

Exchanges: 2 Lean Meat, 1-3/4 Starch, 1 Vegetable

Nutritional Information

Serving Size: 1/6 recipe
Calories: 329
Sodium: 688 mg
Cholesterol: 52 mg

Carbohydrate: 34 gm
Protein: 29 gm
Fat: 8 gm

Grilled Flank Steak

Jenny Reece, Farwell, Minnesota

This recipe is from my sister and it's a favorite of mine for serving company. The meat and vegetables can be prepared ahead of time...when the company arrives, I just fire up the grill and serve a meaty main meal in minutes!

1/4 cup soy sauce
2 tablespoons vinegar
1 green onion, sliced
1-1/2 teaspoons garlic powder
1-1/2 teaspoons ground ginger
3 tablespoons honey
3/4 cup vegetable oil
1 flank steak (1-1/2 pounds)
1 pound fresh mushrooms, sliced
1 green pepper, cut into thin strips
1 yellow *or* sweet red pepper, cut into thin strips
3 carrots, julienned

In a glass baking dish, combine first seven ingredients. Place meat in marinade; cover and refrigerate for 24 hours, turning once. Remove meat and reserve marinade. Grill meat over hot coals until cooked to your preference (about 15 minutes for medium). Meanwhile, in a skillet, saute vegetables in 1/4 cup reserved marinade until tender. Slice meat at an angle into thin strips and serve with vegetables. **Yield:** 5 servings.

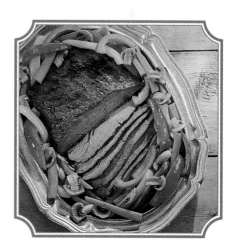

Exchanges: 3 Lean Meat, 2 Vegetable, 1 Fat

Nutritional Information

Serving Size: 1/5 recipe
Calories: 265
Sodium: 173 mg
Cholesterol: 65 mg

Carbohydrate: 11 gm
Protein: 28 gm
Fat: 12 gm

Gone-All-Day Stew

Patty Kile, Plymouth Meeting, Pennsylvania

This healthy, hearty stew is one of my husband's favorite meals. I always use fresh mushrooms, and I toss low-sodium bouillon cubes right into the roaster.

1 can (10-3/4 ounces) condensed tomato soup, undiluted
1 cup water
1/4 cup all-purpose flour
2 pounds beef chuck, fat trimmed, cut into 1-inch to 2-inch cubes
3 medium carrots, cut into 1-inch diagonal slices
6 white boiling onions *or* yellow onions, quartered
4 medium potatoes, cut into 1-1/2-inch chunks
1/2 cup 1-inch celery chunks
12 whole large fresh mushrooms
2 low-sodium beef bouillon cubes
1 tablespoon Italian herb seasoning mix *or* 1 teaspoon *each* leaf oregano, thyme and rosemary
1 bay leaf
3 grinds fresh pepper

Mix together soup, water and flour until smooth; combine with remaining ingredients in covered roasting pan. Bake at 275° for 4-5 hours. Remove bay leaf before serving. **Yield:** 8 servings.

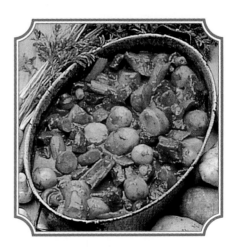

Exchanges: 3 Meat, 2 Vegetable, 1 Starch, 1/2 Fat

Nutritional Information

Serving Size: 1/8 recipe
Calories: 311
Sodium: 441 mg
Cholesterol: 103 mg

Carbohydrate: 26 gm
Protein: 29 gm
Fat: 10 gm

Beef Vegetable Stew

Donna Nannini, Caledonia, Michigan

*Packed with flavorful meat and a huge assortment
of vegetables, this stew is sure to satisfy.*

2-1/2 pounds lean beef stew meat, cut
    into 1-inch cubes
  2 large onions, chopped
  2 garlic cloves, minced
1/2 cup water
  1 low-sodium beef bouillon cube
  6 cups low-sodium beef broth,
    divided
  4 potatoes, peeled and cubed
  3 medium carrots, sliced
  2 medium green peppers, cut into
    1/2-inch pieces
  2 celery ribs, sliced
  3 cups cubed rutabaga
1-1/2 cups cubed parsnips
1-1/2 cups cubed turnips
  3/4 teaspoon dried marjoram

1/2 teaspoon pepper
1/4 teaspoon dried savory
1/4 teaspoon hot pepper sauce
  2 tablespoons cornstarch
  3 tablespoons water

In a Dutch oven, combine the beef, onions, garlic, 1/2 cup water, bouillon and enough of the broth to cover. Bring to a boil. Cover and simmer until meat is tender, about 2 hours. Add vegetables, seasonings and remaining broth. Simmer 30-45 minutes or until vegetables are tender. Combine cornstarch and 3 tablespoons water; gradually add to the boiling mixture. Cook and stir for 2 minutes. **Yield:** 16 servings.

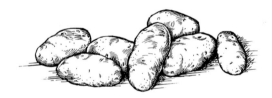

Exchanges: 2 Vegetable, 1 Lean Meat, 1/2 Starch
Nutritional Information
Serving Size: 1 cup
Calories: 143
Sodium: 59 mg
Cholesterol: 21 mg

Carbohydrate: 13 gm
Protein: 15 gm
Fat: 3 gm

Beef Rouladen

Diana Schurrer, McHenry, Illinois

My family came to America from Germany in the late 1950's and brought with them many wonderful recipes like this one. This particular dish reminds me of my grandmother's kitchen and waiting for her delicious dinners.

1 pound thin-cut lean round steak, separated into 4 pieces
Coarse-ground prepared mustard
1/4 teaspoon dried thyme
Pepper to taste
    1 medium dill pickle, quartered lengthwise
    3 carrots, cut into sticks, *divided*
    1 small onion, cut into wedges
    2 tablespoons all-purpose flour
    1 tablespoon cooking oil
    2 cups water
    2 low-sodium beef bouillon cubes
    3 tablespoons ketchup
Hot cooked noodles, optional

Spread steak pieces with mustard. Sprinkle with thyme and pepper. On one edge, place a piece of pickle, carrot and a wedge of onion. Roll up and secure with a toothpick. Coat each roll with flour. In a skillet, heat oil over medium-high. Brown beef on all sides. Add water, bouillon, ketchup and remaining carrots. Cover and simmer for 1 hour. Serve over noodles if desired. **Yield:** 4 servings.

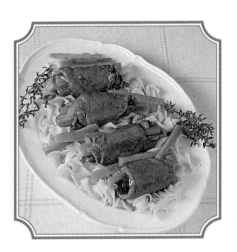

Exchanges: 3 Lean Meat, 1 Vegetable, 1/2 Starch, 1/2 Fat

Nutritional Information

Serving Size: 1/4 recipe
Calories: 250
Sodium: 574 mg
Cholesterol: 70 mg

Carbohydrate: 12 gm
Protein: 26 gm
Fat: 10 gm
(Calculated without noodles)

Shipwreck Stew

Estelle Bates, Fallbrook, California

I got this recipe from a minister's wife, and I imagine she used it many times at church gatherings. It's an inexpensive "stick-to-the-ribs" dinner that's quite easy to prepare. Plus, it tastes even better reheated the next day.

1 pound lean ground beef
1 cup chopped onion
3 cups cubed peeled potatoes
3 medium carrots, sliced
1 cup chopped celery
1/4 cup minced fresh parsley
1 package (9 ounces) frozen cut green beans, defrosted
1 can (15 to 16 ounces) kidney beans, rinsed and drained
1 can (8 ounces) tomato sauce
1/4 cup uncooked long grain rice
1 teaspoon Worcestershire sauce
1/2 to 1 teaspoon chili powder
1/4 teaspoon pepper
1 cup water

In a skillet, brown beef with onion over medium heat. Drain fat. In a 3-qt. casserole, combine beef mixture with all remaining ingredients. Cover and bake at 350° for about 1 hour or until rice and potatoes are tender. **Yield:** 10 servings.

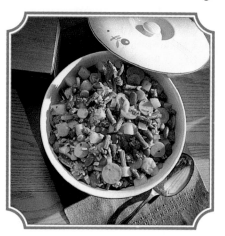

Exchanges: 1-1/2 Lean Meat, 1-1/2 Starch, 1 Vegetable

Nutritional Information

Serving Size: 1/10 recipe
Calories: 204
Sodium: 154 mg
Cholesterol: 32 mg

Carbohydrate: 28 gm
Protein: 15 gm
Fat: 4 gm

Hot Italian Roast Beef Sandwiches

Betty Claycomb, Alverton, Pennsylvania

These sandwiches always make a big hit. The cooking in our area of western Pennsylvania represents a "melting pot" of Italian, Polish and Pennsylvania Dutch (German), so there's a variety of good foods to choose from.

1 tablespoon margarine
1 boneless sirloin tip beef roast
    (5 pounds)
1 can (28 ounces) tomatoes
    with liquid, cut up
1/3 cup water
1 tablespoon ground thyme
1 to 3 teaspoons crushed red
    pepper flakes
Bread *or* rolls of your choice

In a Dutch oven, melt margarine over medium heat. Brown roast on all sides. Add tomatoes, water, thyme and red pepper flakes; cover and simmer until the roast is tender, about 3-1/2 to 4 hours. Add additional water, if necessary, to keep roast simmering in broth. Remove meat from broth and reserve broth. Let the meat stand 20 minutes. Trim any fat and thinly slice meat. When ready to serve, reheat sliced beef in broth. Serve on bread or rolls. **Yield:** 20 servings.

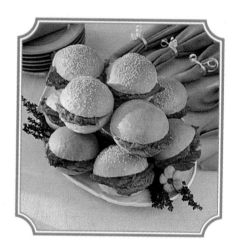

Exchanges: 2 Lean Meat, 1/2 Vegetable

Nutritional Information

Serving Size: 1/20 recipe
Calories: 129
Sodium: 126 mg
Cholesterol: 49 mg

Carbohydrate: 3 gm
Protein: 18 gm
Fat: 5 gm
(Calculated without bread)

Sage Pot Roast

Naomi Giddis, Grawn, Michigan

The addition of sage in this pot roast recipe really adds a unique flavor the whole family will love. Or serve it at your next company dinner. You're sure to get rave reviews!

1 lean boneless beef chuck roast (about 5 pounds)
1 tablespoon cooking oil
1 to 2 teaspoons rubbed sage
1/4 teaspoon pepper
1 cup low-sodium beef broth
6 medium red potatoes (about 2 pounds), cut in half
3 to 4 carrots, cut into 2-inch pieces
2 medium onions, quartered
5 teaspoons cornstarch
1/4 cup water

In a Dutch oven, brown roast on both sides in oil. Season with sage and pepper. Add broth. Cover and bake at 325° for 2-1/2 hours. Add potatoes, carrots and onions. Cover and bake 1 hour longer or until the meat is tender and vegetables are cooked. Remove roast and vegetables to a serving platter and keep warm. Combine cornstarch and water; stir into pan juices. Cook until thickened and bubbly. Serve with the roast. **Yield:** 12 servings.

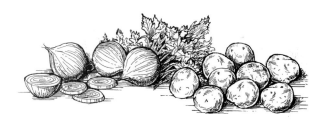

Exchanges: 3 Lean Meat, 1 Starch, 1 Vegetable
Nutritional Information
Serving Size: 1/12 recipe
Calories: 301
Sodium: 59 mg
Cholesterol: 82 mg

Carbohydrate: 16 gm
Protein: 27 gm
Fat: 14 gm

Summary Stuffed Peppers

Pat Whitaker, Lebanon, Oregon

Living in the Willamette Valley of Oregon, we've always had fresh vegetables from the garden, and this recipe allows me to use many of them.

8 medium yellow, green *or* sweet red peppers
1-1/2 pounds lean ground beef
1/2 garlic clove, minced
1 medium onion, minced
1/2 cup finely chopped cabbage
1 medium carrot, shredded
1/2 cup shredded zucchini
1 can (28 ounces) tomatoes with liquid, cut up
1/2 cup uncooked long grain rice
1 tablespoon brown sugar
1/4 teaspoon dried basil
Pepper to taste

Cut the tops off each pepper and reserve. Cook peppers in boiling water until crisp-tender, about 2-3 minutes. Remove from water and rinse with cold water. Remove stems from pepper tops and chop enough of the tops to make 1/3 cup. In a large skillet, brown ground beef over medium heat. Add garlic, onion, cabbage, carrot, zucchini and reserved chopped peppers. Saute until vegetables are tender. Add tomatoes, rice, sugar, basil and pepper. Cover and reduce heat. Simmer until the rice is tender, about 20 minutes. Stuff hot meat mixture into peppers. Serve immediately. **Yield:** 8 servings.

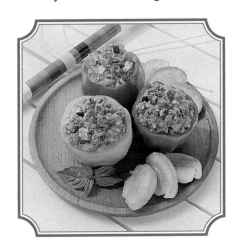

Exchanges: 3 Lean Meat, 2 Vegetable, 1 Starch, 1/2 Fat

Nutritional Information

Serving Size: 1 stuffed pepper
Calories: 315
Sodium: 234 mg
Cholesterol: 67 mg

Carbohydrate: 25 gm
Protein: 28 gm
Fat: 12 gm

Fireside Beef Stew

Donna Nevil, New Glarus, Wisconsin

This stew is perfect for warming up on a wintry day. It's a good dish to make when busy, since it's easy to prepare and doesn't need attention while cooking.

2 pounds lean beef chuck *or* round steak, cut into 1-1/2-inch pieces
1 tablespoon browning sauce
1/4 cup dry cream of rice cereal
4 carrots, cut into 1-1/2-inch chunks
2 cups thinly sliced onion
1 garlic clove, minced
1/2 to 1 teaspoon dried marjoram, crushed
1/2 to 1 teaspoon dried thyme, crushed
1/4 teaspoon pepper
1 cup low-sodium beef broth
1 jar (4-1/2 ounces) button mushrooms, undrained
Hot cooked noodles, optional

In a medium Dutch oven or 3-qt. casserole, toss meat with browning sauce. Mix in cereal. Add all remaining ingredients except noodles. Cover and bake at 325° for 2 to 2-1/2 hours or until the meat and vegetables are tender. Serve over noodles if desired. **Yield:** 8 servings.

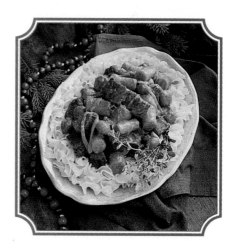

Exchanges: 2 Lean Meat, 1-1/2 Vegetable, 1/2 Starch
Nutritional Information
Serving Size: 1/8 recipe
Calories: 199
Sodium: 50 mg
Cholesterol: 72 mg

Carbohydrate: 12 gm
Protein: 21 gm
Fat: 6 gm
(Calculated without noodles)

Summer's End Stew

Laura Garton, Lenox, Massachusetts

My family loves stew, and this recipe is perfect for the last few vegetables left in the garden.

1-1/2 pounds lean beef stew meat, trimmed
1 tablespoon cooking oil
8 to 12 medium fresh tomatoes, peeled and cut up
2 cups low-sodium tomato juice *or* water
2 medium onions, chopped
1 garlic clove, minced
1/2 teaspoon pepper
4 to 6 medium potatoes, peeled and quartered
3 to 5 carrots, sliced
2 cups frozen corn
2 cups fresh cut green beans
2 cups frozen peas
2 to 3 celery ribs, sliced
1 cup sliced summer squash
1/4 cup snipped fresh parsley
1 teaspoon sugar

In a Dutch oven, brown meat in oil over medium-high heat. Add tomatoes, tomato juice or water, onions, garlic and pepper. Bring to a boil; reduce heat and simmer for 1 hour. Add potatoes, carrots, corn, green beans, peas and celery. Cover and simmer 30 minutes. Add squash; simmer 10-15 minutes or until meat and vegetables are tender. Stir in parsley and sugar. **Yield:** 16 servings.

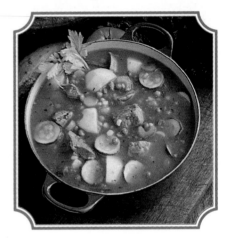

Exchanges: 2 Vegetable, 1 Meat, 1 Starch
Nutritional Information

Serving Size: 1 cup
Calories: 189
Sodium: 170 mg
Cholesterol: 32 mg

Carbohydrate: 22 gm
Protein: 13 gm
Fat: 6 gm

Vegetable Beef Stir-Fry

Cathy Stelbrink, Kampsville, Illinois

With such robust flavor, no one will ever guess this super stir-fry is low in fat! So even folks not on restricted diets will find it appealing.

1 pound ground round
1 medium onion, sliced
2 garlic cloves, minced
1 green pepper, julienned
4 ounces fresh mushrooms, sliced
1 package (16 ounces) frozen
  stir-fry vegetables, thawed
1 can (14 ounces) bean sprouts,
  drained
1 can (8 ounces) sliced water
  chestnuts, drained
1 cup low-sodium beef broth
2 tablespoons cornstarch
1/4 cup light soy sauce
3/4 teaspoon ground ginger

In a large skillet, stir-fry the meat until browned; drain. Add onion and garlic; stir-fry 2 minutes. Add green pepper, mushrooms, vegetables, sprouts and water chestnuts. Stir-fry 3-4 minutes or until crisp-tender. Combine broth, cornstarch, soy sauce and ginger; stir into skillet. Bring to a boil; cook for 1 minute. **Yield:** 8 servings.

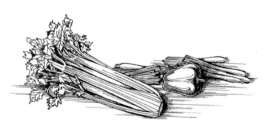

Exchanges: 2 Meat, 2 Vegetable
Nutritional Information

Serving Size: 1 cup
Calories: 202
Sodium: 346 mg
Cholesterol: 38 mg

Carbohydrate: 11 gm
Protein: 16 gm
Fat: 8 gm

French Dip Sandwiches

Dianne Joy Richardson, Colorado Springs, Colorado

This recipe is great for an easy meal, since the meat cooks all day without any attention. Kids of all ages are fond of these super sandwiches.

1 lean beef roast (3 to 4
   pounds)
1/2 cup light soy sauce
1 low-sodium beef bouillon cube
1 bay leaf
3 to 4 whole peppercorns
1 teaspoon dried rosemary, crushed
1 teaspoon dried thyme
1 teaspoon garlic powder
Bread *or* rolls of your choice

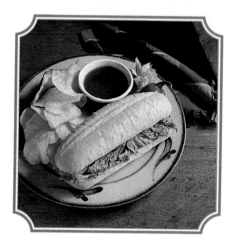

Remove and discard all visible fat from roast. Place in a slow cooker. Combine soy sauce, bouillon and spices; pour over roast. Add water to almost cover roast. Cover and cook over low heat 10-12 hours or until meat is very tender. Remove meat from broth; shred with a fork. Serve on bread or rolls. **Yield:** 12 servings.

Exchanges: 3 Lean Meat
Nutritional Information

Serving Size: 1/12 recipe	Carbohydrate: 1 gm
Calories: 175	Protein: 25 gm
Sodium: 360 mg	Fat: 8 gm
Cholesterol: 69 mg	*(Calculated without bread)*

Steak and Vegetable Kabobs

Lorri Cleveland, Kingsville, Ohio

You can spend the day out of the kitchen by assembling these kabobs in the morning, then letting them marinate all day before grilling at dinnertime.

1/4 cup vegetable oil
1/4 cup lemon juice
1/4 cup soy sauce
1/4 cup packed brown sugar
2 garlic cloves, minced
3 whole cloves
Dash dried sweet basil
2-1/2 pounds sirloin steak, cut into
    1-1/4-inch pieces
2 dozen cherry tomatoes
2 dozen fresh mushroom caps
1 large green *or* sweet red
    pepper, cut into 1-1/2-inch cubes
2 small zucchini, cut into 1-inch
    slices
1 medium onion, cut into wedges
Hot cooked rice, optional

In a bowl, combine first seven ingredients for the marinade. Set aside. Assemble kabobs by threading meat and vegetables on metal skewers. Place in a large glass dish. Pour marinade over kabobs; cover and refrigerate 6 hours or overnight. Turn several times. To cook, grill kabobs over hot coals until the meat and vegetables have reached desired doneness. Remove from the skewers; serve over rice if desired. **Yield:** 10 servings.

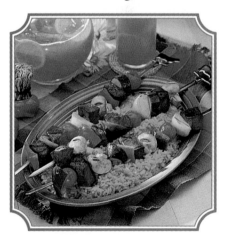

Exchanges: 2 Meat, 1-1/2 Vegetable

Nutritional Information

Serving Size: 1/10 recipe
Calories: 195
Sodium: 381 mg
Cholesterol: 49 mg

Carbohydrate: 8 gm
Protein: 19 gm
Fat: 10 gm
(Calculated without rice)

Marinated Flank Steak

Debbie Bonczek, Tariffville, Connecticut

I copied this recipe from a friend's collection 15 years ago. Whenever we make steak on the grill, this is the recipe we usually use. It's also a tempting dish to serve when entertaining. It's earned me many compliments.

1 flank steak (about 2 pounds)
3 tablespoons ketchup
1 tablespoon vegetable oil
1 tablespoon chopped onion
1 teaspoon brown sugar
1 teaspoon Worcestershire sauce
1 garlic clove, minced
1/8 teaspoon pepper

Place flank steak in an 11-in. x 7-in. x 2-in. glass dish. Combine remaining ingredients; pour over meat. Cover and refrigerate for at least 4 hours. Remove meat, discarding marinade. Grill over hot coals until meat reaches desired doneness, about 4 minutes per side for medium, 5 minutes per side for medium-well. Slice into thin strips across the grain to serve. **Yield:** 8 servings.

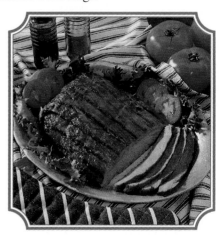

Exchanges: 3 Lean Meat

Nutritional Information

Serving Size: 1/8 recipe
Calories: 172
Sodium: 115 mg
Cholesterol: 43 mg

Carbohydrate: 2 gm
Protein: 23 gm
Fat: 7 gm

Beef Barley Stew

June Formanek, Belle Plaine, Iowa

It's nice to indulge in hearty, down-home dishes without worrying about the fat. That's why I know you and your family will surely savor this stew.

1-1/2 pounds lean beef stew meat, cut
    into 1/2-inch cubes
  1 medium onion, chopped
  1 tablespoon cooking oil
  6 cups low-sodium beef broth
  1 cup medium pearl barley
  1 teaspoon dried thyme
  1/2 teaspoon dried marjoram
  1/4 teaspoon dried rosemary,
    crushed
  1/4 teaspoon pepper
  4 medium carrots, sliced
  2 tablespoons chopped fresh
    parsley

In a large saucepan or Dutch oven over medium heat, brown meat and onion in oil. Add broth, barley, thyme, marjoram, rosemary and pepper; bring to a boil. Reduce heat; cover and simmer for 1 hour. Add carrots; bring to a boil. Reduce heat; cover and simmer 30-40 minutes or until meat and carrots are tender. Add parsley just before serving. **Yield:** 8 servings.

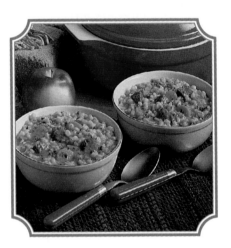

Exchanges: 3 Lean Meat, 1 Starch, 1 Vegetable

Nutritional Information

Serving Size: 1/8 recipe
Calories: 266
Sodium: 618 mg
Cholesterol: 40 mg

Carbohydrate: 24 gm
Protein: 23 gm
Fat: 8 gm

Spicy Tomato Steak

Anne Landers, Louisville, Kentucky

My family loves this spicy tomato dish. I came up with the recipe about 25 years ago, after eating a similar dish on vacation in New Mexico.

2 tablespoons vinegar
1 teaspoon pepper
1 pound round steak, trimmed
  and cut into 1/4-inch strips
1/4 cup all-purpose flour
2 tablespoons olive oil
3 medium tomatoes, peeled,
  cut into wedges and seeded
2 medium potatoes, peeled and
  thinly sliced
2 cans (4 ounces *each*)
  chopped green chilies
1 garlic clove, minced
1 teaspoon dried basil

In a mixing bowl, combine vinegar and pepper; toss with beef. Cover and refrigerate for 30 minutes; drain. Place flour in a bowl; add beef and toss to coat. In a skillet, cook beef in oil over medium heat for 15-20 minutes or until tender. Add remaining ingredients. Cover and simmer for 20-30 minutes or until the potatoes are tender, stirring occasionally. **Yield:** 6 servings.

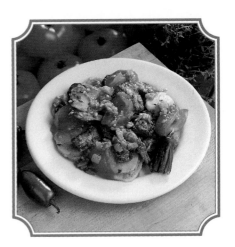

Exchanges: 2 Lean Meat, 1 Starch, 1/2 Fat
Nutritional Information

Serving Size: 1/6 recipe
Calories: 195
Sodium: 364 mg
Cholesterol: 24 mg

Carbohydrate: 16 gm
Protein: 16 gm
Fat: 8 gm

Easy Oven Stew

Carol Smith, Stuart, Florida

Not only is this stew delicious, anybody can make it—you just throw the ingredients into a pot and stir! This dish really lives up to its name.

2 pounds lean beef stew meat, cut into 1-inch cubes
4 large carrots, cut into 1-inch pieces
2 medium onions, cut into 1-inch pieces
2 celery ribs, cut into 1-inch pieces
2 medium parsnips, cut into 1-inch pieces
1 garlic clove, minced
1 can (14-1/2 ounces) Italian stewed tomatoes
1-1/2 cups low-sodium beef broth
1 can (8 ounces) low-sodium tomato sauce
1/2 cup quick-cooking tapioca
1 teaspoon instant coffee granules
1/2 teaspoon dried thyme
1/2 teaspoon dried oregano

In a 5-qt. Dutch oven, combine all ingredients. Cover and bake at 300° for 2-1/2 to 3 hours, stirring every hour, or until the meat and vegetables are tender. **Yield:** 8 servings.

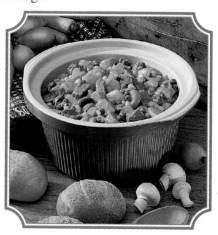

Exchanges: 2 Meat, 2 Vegetable. 1 Starch
Nutritional Information
Serving Size: 1-1/3 cups
Calories: 230
Sodium: 401 mg
Cholesterol: 53 mg

Carbohydrate: 27 gm
Protein: 23 gm
Fat: 6 gm

Hamburger Casserole

Helen Carmichall, Santee, California

This recipe is such a hit it's "traveled" all over the country! My mother originated the recipe in Pennsylvania...I brought it to Texas when I married...I'm still making it in California... and my daughter treats her friends to this "oldie" in Colorado.

2 pounds uncooked extra lean ground beef *or* **ground round**
4 pounds potatoes, peeled and sliced 1/4 inch thick
1 large onion, sliced
1/2 teaspoon pepper
1 low-sodium beef bouillon cube
1 cup hot water
1 can (28 ounces) tomatoes with liquid, cut up
Chopped fresh parsley, optional

In a Dutch oven, layer half of the meat, potatoes and onion. Sprinkle with half of the pepper. Repeat layers. Dissolve bouillon in water; pour over all. Top with tomatoes. Cover and cook over medium heat for 45-50 minutes or until potatoes are tender. Garnish with parsley if desired. **Yield:** 10 servings.

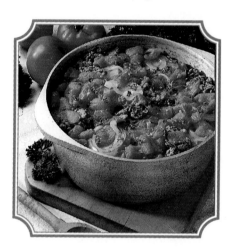

Exchanges: 3 Lean Meat, 2 Starch
Nutritional Information

Serving Size: 1/10 recipe
Calories: 314
Sodium: 189 mg
Cholesterol: 74 mg

Carbohydrate: 33 gm
Protein: 28 gm
Fat: 8 gm

Italian Flank Steak

Walajean Saglett, Canandaigua, New York

*This beef recipe is perfect for entertaining because
it marinates overnight and grills in minutes. Try leftovers—
if there are any—in sandwiches the next day.*

**1 package (1.2 ounces) Italian
salad dressing mix
2 tablespoons vegetable oil
1 tablespoon lemon juice
1 flank steak (1 pound)**

In a small bowl, combine salad dressing, oil and lemon juice. Spread half over one side of steak. Roll up jelly-roll style, with seasoned side in; secure with string and place in a small baking pan. Spread remaining dressing mixture on outside of steak. Cover and refrigerate several hours or overnight. Grill over hot coals for about 15 minutes or until desired doneness is reached, turning frequently. Remove string and lay steak flat on the grill to sear inside for several minutes. **Yield:** 4 servings.

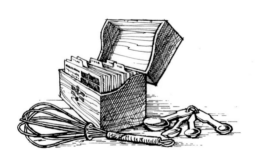

Exchanges: 3 Meat

Nutritional Information

Serving Size: 1/4 recipe
Calories: 214
Sodium: 392 mg
Cholesterol: 60 mg

Carbohydrate: 1 gm
Protein: 22 gm
Fat: 16 gm

Savory Pot Roast

Joan Hutter, Warnick, Rhode Island

I liked it when Grandma made pot roast because she'd let me help. I diced the onions, opened the can of tomatoes and measured out the horseradish. Handling that horseradish always made my eyes tear!

**1 round-bone chuck roast
  (3 pounds)**
1 tablespoon cooking oil
2 large onions, diced
2 garlic cloves, minced
**1 can (16 ounces) tomatoes with
  liquid, cut up**
1 cup water, *divided*
**2 tablespoons prepared
  horseradish**
1 teaspoon browning sauce
1/8 teaspoon pepper

In a Dutch oven, brown roast in oil. Remove and set aside. In the drippings, saute onions and garlic until onions are tender. Return roast to Dutch oven. Stir in tomatoes, 1/2 cup water, horseradish, browning sauce and pepper. Cover and simmer for 2-3 hours or until meat is tender. **Yield:** 8 servings.

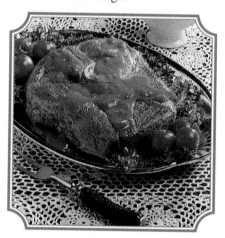

Exchanges: 3 Lean Meat, 1 Fat
Nutritional Information

Serving Size: 1/8 recipe
Calories: 263
Sodium: 121 mg
Cholesterol: 92 mg

Carbohydrate: 4 gm
Protein: 28 gm
Fat: 15 gm

Teriyaki Finger Steaks

Jeri Dobrowski, Beach, North Dakota

When these flavorful skewered steaks are sizzling on the grill, the aroma makes everyone around stop what they're doing and come see what's cooking. The tasty marinade is easy to make, and these little steaks are quick to cook and fun to eat.

2 pounds boneless sirloin steak
1/2 cup light soy sauce
1/4 cup vinegar
2 tablespoons brown sugar
2 tablespoons minced onion
1 tablespoon vegetable oil
1 garlic clove, minced
1/2 teaspoon ground ginger
1/8 teaspoon pepper

Trim fat from steak and slice lengthwise into 1/2-in. strips; place in a large glass bowl. Combine all remaining ingredients; pour over meat and toss gently. Cover and refrigerate for 2-3 hours. Drain, discarding marinade. Loosely thread meat strips onto skewers. Grill over medium-hot coals, turning often, for 7-10 minutes or until meat reaches desired doneness. Remove from skewers and serve. **Yield:** 6 servings.

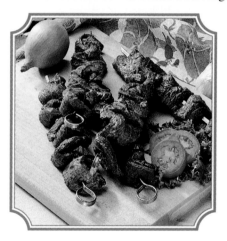

Exchanges: 3 Lean Meat, 1/2 Starch
Nutritional Information

Serving Size: 1/6 recipe
Calories: 190
Sodium: 725 mg
Cholesterol: 62 mg

Carbohydrate: 6 gm
Protein: 24 gm
Fat: 7 gm

One-Dish Oven Stew

Rita Zagrzebski, Eagle River, Wisconsin

I like to keep busy on weekends and don't want to be tied up in the kitchen. That's when this recipe comes in handy. With little fuss, a hearty stew awaits you at the end of the day.

3/4 pound boneless beef round steak, trimmed and cubed
1 tablespoon cooking oil
4 medium unpeeled potatoes, cut into 1-inch cubes
5 medium carrots, cut into 1-1/2-inch chunks
1 celery rib, cut into 1-inch chunks
1 large onion, cut into 1-inch chunks
1 can (14-1/2 ounces) chunky stewed tomatoes
3 tablespoons quick-cooking tapioca
1 teaspoon browning sauce
1/8 to 1/4 teaspoon pepper
1 cup frozen peas

In a Dutch oven, brown the steak in oil. Add the next eight ingredients; cover and bake at 300° for 4-5 hours, stirring twice. Add the peas during the last 30 minutes of baking. **Yield:** 6 servings.

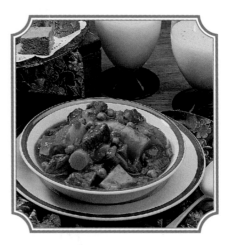

Italian Shepherd's Pie

Rosanne Reynolds, Kissimmee, Florida

*You just can't beat the convenience of this one-dish meal.
I often prepare this pie the night before so that the next day,
I can serve my family a satisfying meal in no time.*

1 cup Italian bread crumbs
1 cup cold water
4 medium potatoes, peeled
1-1/4 pounds uncooked ground round
1/2 cup finely chopped onion
1/2 cup finely chopped celery
1 can (8 ounces) tomato sauce
1 can (4 ounces) mushrooms,
  drained and finely chopped
1 garlic clove, minced
1/4 teaspoon pepper
1-1/2 cups frozen peas and carrots
1/2 cup shredded low-fat
  mozzarella cheese

Combine crumbs and water; let stand for 5 minutes. Cook potatoes in boiling water until tender. Meanwhile, combine meat, onion, celery, tomato sauce, mushrooms, garlic and pepper. Stir in crumb mixture. Spread into an ungreased 11-in. x 7-in. x 2-in. baking dish. Top with peas and carrots. Drain the potatoes; mash with cheese. Spread over vegetables, sealing to pan. Bake at 375° for 45-60 minutes. **Yield:** 6 servings.

DINNER FOR TWO? When cooking for one or two people, divide casserole ingredients into two smaller dishes and freeze one for later use. You'll appreciate the ready-to-make meal on busy days.

Exchanges: 3-1/2 Lean Meat, 2-1/2 Starch, 1 Vegetable

Nutritional Information

Serving Size: 1/6 recipe
Calories: 398
Sodium: 976 mg
Cholesterol: 80 mg

Carbohydrate: 43 gm
Protein: 34 gm
Fat: 11 gm

Salisbury Steak

Carol Callahan, Rome, Georgia

This meat dish can be made in 25 minutes, or made ahead and reheated with the gravy in the microwave. After one bite, I think you and your family will agree Salisbury Steak never tasted so good!

1 pound lean ground beef
1 egg white, lightly beaten
1/3 cup chopped onion
1/4 cup saltine crumbs
2 tablespoons skim milk
1 tablespoon prepared horseradish
1/8 teaspoon pepper
1 jar (12 ounces) low-fat beef gravy
1-1/4 to 1-1/2 cups sliced fresh mushrooms
2 tablespoons water
Hot cooked noodles, optional

In a bowl, combine the beef, egg white, onion, crumbs, milk, horseradish and pepper. Shape into four oval patties. Fry in a skillet over medium heat for 10-12 minutes or until cooked through, turning once.

Remove patties and keep warm. Add gravy, mushrooms and water to skillet; heat for 3-5 minutes. Serve over patties and noodles if desired. **Yield:** 4 servings.

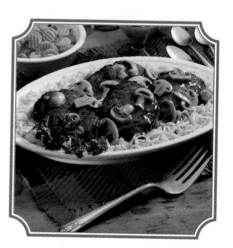

Exchanges: 3 Meat, 1/2 Starch, 1/2 Vegetable

Nutritional Information

Serving Size: 1/4 recipe
Calories: 248
Sodium: 205 mg
Cholesterol: 66 mg

Carbohydrate: 9 gm
Protein: 25 gm
Fat: 12 gm
(Calculated without noodles)

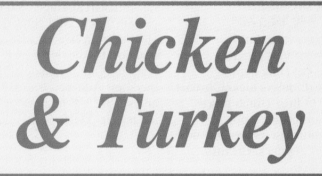

Chicken
& Turkey

*When your mouth-watering menu features
fantastic fowl, the meal is guaranteed
to be an astounding success.*

Chicken 'n' Peppers

Cathy Zoller, Lovell, Wyoming

With garden-fresh peppers and tender chicken, this dish is perfect when your family is craving a lighter dinner. I like to serve it with rice and a green salad.

3/4 cup low-sodium chicken broth
1/4 cup light soy sauce
2 garlic cloves, minced
2 tablespoons cornstarch
3/4 teaspoon ground ginger
1/4 teaspoon cayenne pepper
6 boneless skinless chicken breast halves, cut into 1-inch pieces
1 tablespoon cooking oil
1 *each* medium green, yellow and sweet red peppers, cut into 1-inch pieces
1/4 cup water

In a bowl, combine broth, soy sauce, garlic, cornstarch, ginger and cayenne pepper; mix well. Add chicken; stir to coat. Heat oil in a large skillet over medium-high heat. Add chicken; cook and stir constantly for 7 minutes. Reduce heat to medium. Add peppers and water; cook and stir for 5-8 minutes or until peppers are tender. **Yield:** 6 servings.

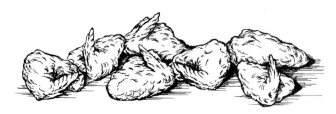

Exchanges: 3 Lean Meat, 1 Vegetable
Nutritional Information

Serving Size: 1/6 recipe
Calories: 200
Sodium: 207 mg
Cholesterol: 73 mg

Carbohydrate: 8 gm
Protein: 29 gm
Fat: 7 gm

Meaty Spanish Rice

Margaret Shauers, Great Bend, Kansas

I usually fix this slightly spicy rice for family meals—but it's also great for doubling if unexpected company comes and the cupboards are all nearly bare! It's always a hit whenever I make it.

2 tablespoons margarine
1/2 pound ground turkey
1 medium onion, chopped
1 medium green pepper, chopped
2 cups water
1 can (8 ounces) tomato sauce
1 cup uncooked long grain rice
2 tablespoons Worcestershire sauce
1/2 teaspoon chili powder
1/2 teaspoon dried thyme
1/4 teaspoon hot pepper sauce
1/8 teaspoon cayenne pepper, optional
Pepper to taste

In a skillet, melt margarine over medium heat. Add turkey, onion and green pepper; cook until meat is browned and vegetables are tender. Add remaining ingredients and bring to a boil. Reduce heat; cover and simmer until rice is tender, about 30 minutes. **Yield:** 4 servings.

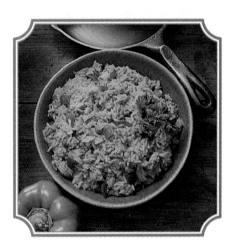

Exchanges: 2 Meat, 1-3/4 Starch, 1 Fat

Nutritional Information

Serving Size: 1/4 recipe
Calories: 300
Sodium: 379 mg
Cholesterol: 52 mg

Carbohydrate: 27 gm
Protein: 17 gm
Fat: 14 gm

Chicken Mushroom Stir-Fry

Christina Thompson, Howell, Michigan

When I had co-workers sample this recipe, the dish ended up empty!

1 tablespoon light soy sauce
1 egg white
1 teaspoon sesame oil
1/2 teaspoon brown sugar
1 teaspoon cornstarch
1/8 teaspoon white pepper
1 pound boneless skinless chicken
  breasts, cut into 1/2-inch cubes
1/2 cup low-sodium chicken broth
2 tablespoons cornstarch
2 tablespoons cold water
1/4 cup oyster sauce
4 tablespoons vegetable oil, *divided*
1-1/2 teaspoons minced fresh
  gingerroot
2 garlic cloves, minced
2 green onions, sliced
4 medium carrots, cubed
1 pound fresh mushrooms,
  quartered
1/4 pound fresh snow peas, trimmed
  and halved

Combine first six ingredients; toss with chicken. Refrigerate 30 minutes. In a small bowl, combine chicken broth, cornstarch, water and oyster sauce. Set aside. In a wok or large skillet, heat 2 tablespoons oil over medium-high. Add gingerroot, garlic and onions; stir-fry 1 minute. Add chicken and continue to stir-fry until the chicken is no longer pink. Remove chicken and vegetables from pan. Add remaining oil; stir-fry carrots 3 minutes or until crisp-tender. Add mushrooms and peas; stir-fry 1 minute. Return chicken and vegetables to pan. Stir broth mixture and pour into skillet; cook and stir until the sauce is thickened. Serve immediately. **Yield:** 6 servings.

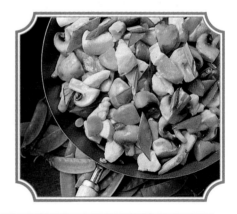

Exchanges: 3 Lean Meat, 1 Vegetable, 1 Fat, 3/4 Starch

Nutritional Information

Serving Size: 1/6 recipe
Calories: 299
Sodium: 431 mg
Cholesterol: 68 mg

Carbohydrate: 15 gm
Protein: 30 gm
Fat: 14 gm

Chicken and Dumplings

Patricia Collins, Imbler, Oregon

This is so easy and filling...you can fix it anytime. Sometimes, I'll prepare the chicken the day before. Then, when we get home, I'll reheat it, mix up my dumplings, plop them on top and have supper ready in 20 minutes.

1 broiler-fryer chicken (3 pounds), cut up
3 cups water
1 cup chopped onion
4 celery ribs, sliced
3 carrots, sliced
1 teaspoon celery seed
2 teaspoons sage, *divided*
1/4 teaspoon pepper
3 cups baking mix
3/4 cup plus 2 tablespoons milk
1 tablespoon minced fresh parsley

Place chicken and water in a Dutch oven. Cover and bring to a boil. Reduce heat; simmer until chicken is tender, about 30-45 minutes. Remove chicken; bone and cube. Skim fat; return chicken to kettle along with onion, celery, carrots, celery seed, 1 teaspoon of sage and pepper. Cover and simmer for 45-60 minutes or until the vegetables are tender. For dumplings, combine baking mix, milk, parsley and remaining sage to form a stiff batter. Drop by tablespoonfuls into the simmering chicken mixture. Cover and simmer for 15 minutes. Serve immediately. **Yield:** 8 servings.

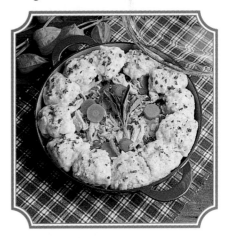

Exchanges: 2 Starch, 2 Meat
Nutritional Information

Serving Size: 1/8 recipe
Calories: 276
Sodium: 284 mg
Cholesterol: 29 mg

Carbohydrate: 30 gm
Protein: 20 gm
Fat: 9 gm

Stuffed Chicken Breasts

Jamie Harris, Bodega, California

More than at any other time of year, watching your diet around the holidays can be a real challenge. That's when I reach for this chicken recipe. It's festive and full-flavored, so you won't feel like you're missing out on the best tastes of the season.

4 boneless skinless chicken
   breast halves
1/2 cup diced fresh mushrooms
1/2 cup diced green pepper
1/4 cup diced onion
3 garlic cloves, minced
1/4 cup low-sodium vegetable *or*
   chicken broth
1 cup cooked rice
2 cups crushed cornflakes
1/2 teaspoon garlic powder
1/8 teaspoon cayenne pepper
1 cup skim milk

Pound chicken breasts to 1/4-in. thickness and set aside. In a saucepan, combine mushrooms, green pepper, onion, garlic and broth; bring to a boil. Reduce heat and simmer 3 minutes. Remove from the heat; add rice. Mix well and set aside. Combine cornflakes, garlic powder and cayenne pepper; mix well. Set aside. Spoon a fourth of the rice mixture onto the center of each chicken breast. Fold chicken around rice mixture; seal with toothpicks. Dip chicken in milk. Coat all sides with cornflake mixture. Place chicken in a shallow baking dish that has been coated with nonstick cooking spray. Spray tops of chicken with cooking spray. Bake at 375° for 55-60 minutes or until juices run clear. **Yield:** 4 servings.

Exchanges: 3 Starch, 3 Lean Meat, 1 Vegetable
Nutritional Information

Serving Size: 1 chicken
breast half
Calories: 399
Sodium: 572 mg

Cholesterol: 74 mg
Carbohydrate: 55 gm
Protein: 34 gm
Fat: 4 gm

Chicken and Apricot Saute

Carolyn Griffin, Macon, Georgia

This is a popular dish in our home. The combination of chicken and slightly sweet apricots tastes good, and stir-frying is a method of cooking I really enjoy. It's a quick and healthy way to prepare food, too!

1 cup low-sodium chicken broth
1 tablespoon cornstarch
Pepper to taste
1 tablespoon cooking oil
1 pound boneless skinless chicken breasts, cut into thin strips
3 cups sliced celery
2 garlic cloves, minced
1 can (16 ounces) apricot halves in natural juices, drained
6 ounces fresh *or* frozen snow peas

Combine broth, cornstarch and pepper. Set aside. In a wok or large skillet, heat oil on high. Add chicken; stir-fry until no longer pink. Remove from pan. Add celery and garlic; stir-fry until the celery is crisp-tender, about 3 minutes. Stir in broth mixture. Cook, stirring constantly until thick, about 1 minute. Add apricots, peas and cooked chicken. Stir-fry until heated through, about 1-2 minutes. **Yield:** 6 servings.

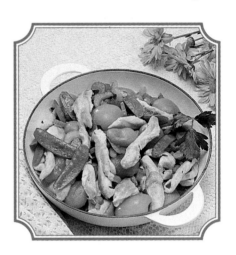

Exchanges: 2-1/2 Lean Meat, 1-1/2 Vegetable, 1/2 Fruit

Nutritional Information

Serving Size: 1/6 recipe
Calories: 204
Sodium: 114 mg
Cholesterol: 64 mg

Carbohydrate: 14 gm
Protein: 25 gm
Fat: 5 gm

Chicken Cacciatore

Emily Nieves, Wildomar, California

This recipe has been in my family for a long time. I remember my grandmother making it on special occasions. In those days, chicken was a treat, and we relished every bite—especially if Grandmother cooked it!

1 cup all-purpose flour
2 broiler-fryer chickens (about 2-1/2 pounds *each*), cut up
3 tablespoons olive oil
3 garlic cloves, minced
2 medium onions, chopped
1/2 pound fresh mushrooms, sliced
1 cup low-sodium chicken broth
2 cups canned tomato puree
1 teaspoon dried oregano
1/4 cup chopped fresh parsley
1/8 teaspoon pepper
Cooked pasta, optional

Place flour in a bag; shake chicken, a few pieces at a time, to coat. In a large skillet, heat oil over medium-high. Brown chicken on all sides. Remove chicken and set aside. In the skillet, saute garlic and onions until onions are soft. Add mushrooms, broth, tomato puree, oregano, parsley and pepper; bring to a boil. Return chicken to skillet; cover and simmer 1 hour or until chicken is tender. Serve over pasta if desired. **Yield:** 8 servings.

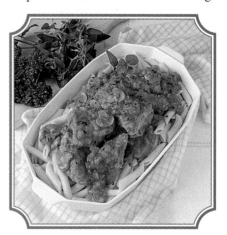

Exchanges: 4 Lean Meat, 2 Vegetable, 1 Starch, 1/2 Fat

Nutritional Information

Serving Size: 1/8 recipe
Calories: 402
Sodium: 33 mg
Cholesterol: 91 mg

Carbohydrate: 26 gm
Protein: 39 gm
Fat: 15 gm
(Calculated without pasta)

Basil Chicken Medley

Susan Jansen, Smyrna, Georgia

Everyone who's tried this dish has raved about it. I came up with this quick, colorful main course right in my own kitchen. It's easy to put together when time is scarce.

1 tablespoon olive oil
3 garlic cloves, minced
2 whole boneless skinless chicken breasts (about 1-1/4 pounds), cut into 1-inch chunks
1 medium zucchini, cut into chunks
2 medium tomatoes, cut into chunks
2 tablespoons vinegar

1 tablespoon dried basil
1/4 teaspoon pepper

Heat oil in a skillet; saute garlic. Add chicken and cook until no longer pink; remove and keep warm. Combine zucchini, tomatoes, vinegar, basil and pepper; toss to coat vegetables well. Add to skillet and stir-fry about 3-5 minutes. Return chicken to skillet and heat through. **Yield:** 4 servings.

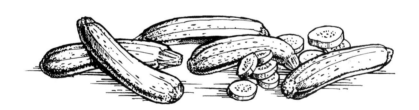

Exchanges: 3 Lean Meat, 1 Vegetable

Nutritional Information

Serving Size: 1/4 recipe
Calories: 205
Sodium: 70 mg
Cholesterol: 73 mg

Carbohydrate: 8 gm
Protein: 28 gm
Fat: 7 gm

Chicken Angelo

Carol Oswald, Schnecksville, Pennsylvania

My grandmother always made this dish when we came over for Sunday dinner. I still enjoy it today—it's quick and simple, and I can garden while it cooks!

8 ounces fresh mushrooms,
   sliced, *divided*
4 large boneless skinless chicken
   breast halves
Egg substitute equivalent to 2 eggs
   1 cup bread crumbs
   2 tablespoons margarine
   6 ounces sliced low-fat mozzarella
   cheese
   3/4 cup low-sodium chicken broth
Hot cooked noodles, optional
Chopped fresh parsley

Place half the mushrooms in a 13-in. x 9-in. x 2-in. baking pan. Dip chicken into egg substitute; roll in crumbs. In a skillet, melt margarine over medium heat. Brown chicken on both sides; place on top of mushrooms. Arrange remaining mushrooms over chicken; top with cheese. Add broth to pan. Bake at 350° for 30-35 minutes. Serve over noodles if desired; sprinkle with parsley. **Yield:** 4 servings.

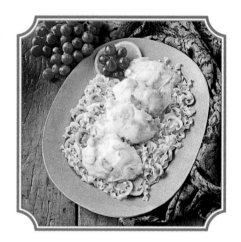

Exchanges: 6 Lean Meat, 1-1/2 Starch, 1 Vegetable

Nutritional Information

Serving Size: 1/4 recipe
Calories: 469
Sodium: 563 mg
Cholesterol: 98 mg

Carbohydrate: 23 gm
Protein: 45 gm
Fat: 21 gm
(Calculated without noodles)

Turkey Legs with Mushroom Gravy

Wanda Swenson, Lady Lake, Florida

Whenever we had company—which was quite often—this dish was a sure hit. We farmed 20 acres for 30 years, so we had plenty of fruits and vegetables on hand to complement this family favorite.

4 turkey legs (about 12 ounces *each*)
1/4 cup lemon juice
2 tablespoons vegetable oil
1 teaspoon dried oregano
1 teaspoon dried basil
1 teaspoon garlic powder
1/4 teaspoon pepper
MUSHROOM GRAVY:
1 cup water
1 tablespoon cornstarch
1 can (4 ounces) sliced mushrooms, drained
1 can (10-1/2 ounces) mushroom gravy
1 teaspoon minced onion
1 tablespoon minced fresh parsley
1 teaspoon garlic powder
Hot cooked noodles, optional

Place turkey legs in a roasting pan. Combine lemon juice, oil and seasonings; pour over turkey. Bake, uncovered, at 375° for 45 minutes or until lightly browned. Turn legs twice and baste occasionally. For gravy, combine water and cornstarch in a saucepan. Stir in mushrooms, gravy, onion, parsley and garlic powder; bring to a boil over medium heat. Spoon over turkey. Cover loosely with foil. Bake, basting frequently, for 1 hour longer or until meat is tender. Serve over noodles if desired. **Yield:** 4 servings.

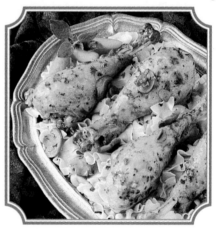

Exchanges: 4 Lean Meat, 1 Vegetable, 1/2 Starch
Nutritional Information
Serving Size: 1/4 recipe
Calories: 270
Sodium: 464 mg
Cholesterol: 132 mg
Carbohydrate: 9 gm
Protein: 35 gm
Fat: 11 gm
(Calculated without noodles)

Grilled Tarragon Chicken

Janie Thorpe, Tullahoma, Tennessee

*We love to grill year-round, and this is one of our favorite recipes.
It's perfect for entertaining because you can spread the chicken with
mustard, refrigerate a few hours and pop on the grill when ready to eat.*

2 teaspoons Dijon mustard
4 boneless skinless chicken breast
  halves
1/4 teaspoon pepper
1/3 cup margarine, melted
2 teaspoons lemon juice
2 teaspoons minced fresh tarragon
  or 1/2 teaspoon dried tarragon
1/2 teaspoon garlic salt

Spread mustard on both sides of chicken; sprinkle with pepper. Cover and refrigerate at least 2 hours. Combine margarine, lemon juice, tarragon and garlic salt. Grill chicken over hot coals until juices run clear, basting with margarine mixture during the last 3-5 minutes. **Yield:** 4 servings.

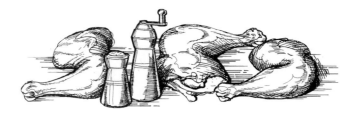

Exchanges: 4 Lean Meat

Nutritional Information

Serving Size: 1 chicken
breast half
Calories: 222
Sodium: 167 mg

Cholesterol: 73 mg
Carbohydrate: 1 gm
Protein: 27 gm
Fat: 12 gm

Baked Chicken Breasts Supreme

Marjorie Scott, Sardis, British Columbia

Perfect for a busy day, this savory main dish can be prepared a day ahead and baked before serving. My brothers don't want me to make anything else when they come to dinner! Leftovers are great, too.

1-1/2 cups plain low-fat yogurt
1/4 cup lemon juice
1/2 teaspoon Worcestershire sauce
1/2 teaspoon celery seed
1/2 teaspoon Hungarian sweet
   paprika
1 garlic clove, minced
1/4 teaspoon pepper
8 boneless skinless chicken
   breast halves
2 cups fine dry bread crumbs

In a large bowl, combine first seven ingredients. Place chicken in mixture and turn to coat. Cover and marinate overnight in the refrigerator. Remove chicken from marinade; coat each piece with crumbs. Arrange on an ungreased shallow baking pan. Bake, uncovered, at 350° for 45 minutes or until juices run clear. **Yield:** 8 servings.

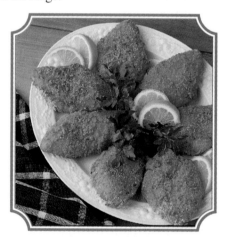

Exchanges: 3-1/2 Lean Meat, 1 Starch, 1/4 Skim Milk

Nutritional Information

Serving Size: 1 chicken
breast half
Calories: 271
Sodium: 293 mg

Cholesterol: 76 mg
Carbohydrate: 22 gm
Protein: 32 gm
Fat: 5 gm

Barbecued Chicken

Joanne Shew Chuk, St. Benedict, Saskatchewan

If you're like me, you can never have enough delicious ways to grill chicken. The savory sauce in this recipe gives the chicken a wonderful herb flavor. It's easy to put together a great meal when you start with these juicy golden pieces.

1 broiler-fryer chicken (3-1/2 pounds), quartered
1/4 cup vinegar
1/4 cup margarine
1/4 cup water
1/4 teaspoon *each* dried thyme, oregano and garlic powder
1/4 teaspoon dried rosemary, crushed
1/8 teaspoon salt
1/8 teaspoon pepper

Place chicken in a shallow glass dish. In a small saucepan, combine all remaining ingredients; bring to a gentle boil. Remove from the heat. Pour over chicken. Cover and refrigerate for 4 hours, turning once. Drain and discard marinade. Grill chicken, covered, over medium coals for 30-40 minutes or until juices run clear. *Remove skin before serving.* **Yield:** 4 servings.

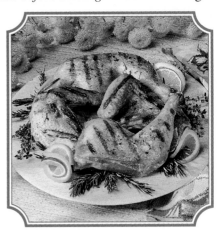

Exchanges: 3 Meat
Nutritional Information

Serving Size: 1/4 recipe
Calories: 224
Sodium: 225 mg
Cholesterol: 58 mg

Carbohydrate: 1 gm
Protein: 21 gm
Fat: 14 gm

Rosemary Chicken

Kathy Anderson, Brookfield, Wisconsin

*Impress friends and family with this simple yet elegant entree.
One taste will have folks requesting the recipe.
You'll want to add it to your family's daily fare, too!*

1 can (14-1/2 ounces) low-sodium chicken broth, *divided*
3 garlic cloves, minced
1 tablespoon finely chopped fresh rosemary *or* 1 teaspoon crushed dried rosemary
1 tablespoon vegetable oil
1 tablespoon light soy sauce
1 teaspoon sugar
1/2 teaspoon pepper
6 boneless skinless chicken breast halves
1 cup uncooked long grain rice
1/2 cup water
10 asparagus spears, blanched and cut into pieces
1 teaspoon grated lemon peel
1 teaspoon lemon-pepper seasoning

In a shallow glass baking dish, combine 1/4 cup broth, garlic, rosemary, oil, soy sauce, sugar and pepper. Add chicken; turn to coat. Cover and refrigerate at least 1 hour. In a saucepan, cook rice in water and remaining broth until soft and fluffy, about 20 minutes. Meanwhile, in a skillet, cook chicken in marinade over medium-high heat for about 7 minutes per side or until chicken is brown and juices run clear. Remove rice from the heat; add asparagus, lemon peel and lemon pepper. Spoon onto individual plates. Cut chicken into strips; arrange in a fan shape over rice. **Yield:** 6 servings.

Exchanges: 3 Lean Meat, 3 Starch
Nutritional Information

Serving Size: 1/6 recipe
Calories: 297
Sodium: 165 mg
Cholesterol: 73 mg

Carbohydrate: 29 gm
Protein: 31 gm
Fat: 8 gm

Spinach Chicken Enchiladas

Joy Headley, Grand Prairie, Texas

My husband is a pastor, so I fix meals for large groups often.
This one is a favorite, and a nice change from the usual beef enchiladas.

4 boneless skinless chicken breast halves, cut into thin strips
1/4 cup chopped onion
1 package (10 ounces) frozen chopped spinach, thawed and well drained
1 can (10-3/4 ounces) condensed low-fat cream of mushroom soup, undiluted
3/4 cup skim milk
1 cup (8 ounces) light sour cream
1 teaspoon ground nutmeg
1 teaspoon garlic powder
1 teaspoon onion powder
8 flour tortillas (8 inches)
2 cups (8 ounces) shredded low-fat mozzarella cheese
Minced fresh parsley

Coat a large skillet with nonstick cooking spray; cook and stir chicken and onion over medium heat for 6-8 minutes or until chicken is no longer pink. Remove from the heat; add spinach and mix well. In a bowl, combine soup, milk, sour cream and seasonings; mix well. Stir 3/4 cup into chicken and spinach mixture. Divide evenly among tortillas. Roll up and place, seam side down, in a 13-in. x 9-in. x 2-in. baking pan that has been sprayed with nonstick cooking spray. Pour the remaining soup mixture over enchiladas. Cover and bake at 350° for 30 minutes. Uncover and sprinkle with cheese; return to the oven for 15 minutes or until cheese is melted and bubbly. Garnish with parsley. **Yield:** 8 servings.

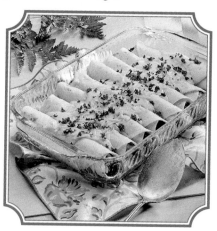

Exchanges: 3 Lean Meat, 1 Vegetable, 1/2 Fat

Nutritional Information

Serving Size: 1 enchilada
Calories: 295
Sodium: 496 mg
Cholesterol: 58 mg

Carbohydrate: 22 gm
Protein: 29 gm
Fat: 11 gm

Zesty Turkey

Rachel Miller, Dodge Center, Minnesota

I frequently prepare this recipe when my family's asking for turkey and when I don't feel like making a whole bird. It's a nice comforting meal for cool fall evenings.

2 tablespoons rubbed sage
1 tablespoon pepper
2 teaspoons curry powder
2 teaspoons garlic powder
2 teaspoons dried parsley flakes
2 teaspoons celery seed
1 teaspoon paprika
1/2 teaspoon dry mustard
1/4 teaspoon ground allspice

3 to 4 bay leaves, crumbled
1 turkey breast (4-1/2 pounds)
2 cups low-sodium chicken broth

In a small bowl, combine spices and mix well. Place turkey on a rack in a roasting pan; rub with spice mixture. Add broth to pan. Bake, uncovered, at 350° for 2-3 hours or until thermometer reads 170°, basting every 30 minutes. **Yield:** 6 servings.

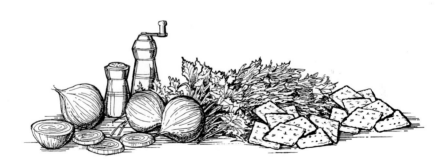

Exchanges: 3-1/2 Lean Meat

Nutritional Information

Serving Size: 1/6 recipe
Calories: 187
Sodium: 85 mg
Cholesterol: 69 mg

Carbohydrate: 3 gm
Protein: 32 gm
Fat: 4 gm

Chicken Fajitas

Lindsay St. John, Plainfield, Indiana

Fajitas are great for those evenings when you want to serve something fun and tasty, yet keep cooking to a minimum.

1/4 cup lime juice
1 garlic clove, minced
1 teaspoon chili powder
1/2 teaspoon ground cumin
2 whole boneless skinless chicken breasts, cut into strips
1 medium onion, cut into thin wedges
1/2 medium sweet red pepper, cut into strips
1/2 medium yellow pepper, cut into strips
1/2 medium green pepper, cut into strips
1/2 cup salsa
12 flour tortillas (8 inches)
1-1/2 cups (6 ounces) shredded low-fat cheddar cheese

In a small bowl, combine lime juice, garlic, chili powder and cumin. Add chicken; stir. Refrigerate for 15 minutes. In a nonstick skillet, cook onion, chicken and marinade for 3 minutes or until chicken is no longer pink. Add peppers; saute for 3-5 minutes or until crisp-tender. Stir in salsa. Divide mixture among tortillas; top with cheese. Roll up and serve. **Yield:** 6 servings.

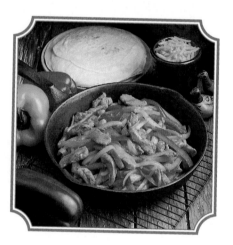

Exchanges: 2 Meat, 1 Vegetable, 1 Starch

Nutritional Information

Serving Size: 2 fajitas
Calories: 228
Sodium: 353 mg
Cholesterol: 39 mg

Carbohydrate: 19 gm
Protein: 17 gm
Fat: 12 gm

Turkey Sausage Stew

Sharon Moon, Hartsville, South Carolina

My family loves traditional beef stew, so they were skeptical when I served this turkey sausage version. But they soon began asking for this stew often.

1 package (16 ounces) frozen
  vegetables for stew
1 can (10-3/4 ounces) condensed
  low-fat tomato soup, undiluted
2 cups water
1 pound low-fat smoked turkey
  sausage, sliced 1/4 inch thick
1/4 cup ketchup

2 garlic cloves, minced
1/2 teaspoon dried basil
1/4 teaspoon pepper

In a large saucepan, combine vegetables, soup and water; bring to a boil. Reduce heat. Add remaining ingredients; simmer for 35-45 minutes or until the vegetables are tender. **Yield:** 8 servings.

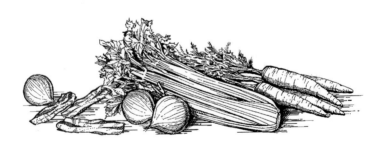

Exchanges: 1-1/2 Meat, 1 Starch

Nutritional Information

Serving Size: 1/8 recipe
Calories: 190
Sodium: 622 mg
Cholesterol: 25 mg

Carbohydrate: 17 gm
Protein: 11 gm
Fat: 8 gm

Dilly Barbecued Turkey

Sue Walker, Greentown, Indiana

*This is one of my brother-in-law's special cookout recipes.
The onions, garlic and herbs in the marinade give the turkey delicious flavor,
and the tempting aroma prompts the family to gather around the grill.*

**1 turkey breast half with bone
(2-1/2 pounds)**
1 cup plain fat-free yogurt
1/4 cup lemon juice
3 tablespoons vegetable oil
1/4 cup minced fresh parsley
1/4 cup chopped green onions
2 garlic cloves, minced
2 tablespoons fresh minced dill
***or* 2 teaspoons dill weed**
**1/2 teaspoon dried rosemary,
crushed**
1/4 teaspoon pepper

Place turkey in a glass baking dish. In a small bowl, combine all remaining ingredients; spread over the turkey. Cover and refrigerate for 6-8 hours or overnight. Remove turkey, reserving marinade. Grill turkey, covered, over medium-hot coals, basting often with marinade, for 1 to 1-1/4 hours or until juices run clear or internal temperature reaches 170°. **Yield:** 6 servings.

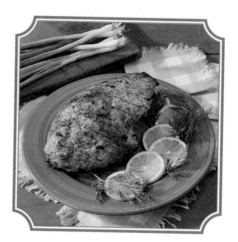

Exchanges: 3 Lean Meat, 1 Vegetable, 1 Fat
Nutritional Information
Serving Size: 1/6 recipe
Calories: 245
Sodium: 127 mg
Cholesterol: 40 mg
Carbohydrate: 5 gm
Protein: 28 gm
Fat: 12 gm

Turkey Stir-Fry

Julianne Johnson, Grove City, Minnesota

My family loves these tender turkey strips and colorful vegetables anytime of year. This recipe proves you don't always have to fix the whole bird to enjoy the wonderful taste of turkey.

1-1/2 pounds uncooked boneless
    turkey breast, cut into strips
1 tablespoon cooking oil
1 small onion, chopped
1 carrot, julienned
1/2 medium green pepper, sliced
2 cups fresh mushrooms, sliced
1 cup low-sodium chicken broth
3 tablespoons cornstarch
3 tablespoons light soy sauce
1/2 teaspoon ground ginger
2 cups fresh snow peas, trimmed

In a large skillet or wok, stir-fry turkey in oil over medium-high heat until no longer pink, about 5-6 minutes. Remove turkey and keep warm. Stir-fry the onion, carrot, green pepper and mushrooms until crisp-tender, about 5 minutes. In a small bowl, combine chicken broth, cornstarch, soy sauce and ginger. Add to the skillet; cook and stir until thickened and bubbly. Return turkey to skillet with peas; cook and stir until heated through. **Yield:** 6 servings.

FOR CRISPIER COLESLAW, cut cabbage heads instead of grating them. Cut cabbage paper-thin with a slicing knife or mechanical shredder. The resulting pieces have more form and the cabbage stays crunchier.

Exchanges: 4 Lean Meat, 1 Vegetable, 1/2 Starch
Nutritional Information
Serving Size: 1/6 recipe
Calories: 277
Sodium: 200 mg
Cholesterol: 84 mg

Carbohydrate: 11 gm
Protein: 40 gm
Fat: 7 gm

Herbed Stuffed Green Peppers

Bea Taus, Fremont, California

*These peppers have a wonderful fresh garden taste.
The herbs add flavor—no need for salt. I like to
serve them with green salad, French bread and fresh fruit.*

6 medium green peppers, tops and seeds removed
1 pound ground turkey breast
1 can (28 ounces) tomatoes with liquid, chopped
1 medium onion, chopped
2 celery ribs, chopped
2 garlic cloves, minced
1 teaspoon dried oregano
1/2 teaspoon dried thyme
1/2 teaspoon dried rosemary, crushed
1/2 teaspoon dried basil
1/2 teaspoon rubbed sage
1/8 teaspoon pepper
1-1/2 cups cooked rice (prepared without salt)
1/3 cup shredded low-fat mozzarella cheese

In a large kettle, blanch peppers in boiling water 3 minutes. Drain and rinse in cold water. Set aside. In a large skillet with a nonstick finish, brown the turkey. Remove and set aside. In the same skillet, combine tomato liquid, onion, celery, garlic and herbs. Simmer until vegetables are tender and the mixture has begun to thicken. Stir in tomatoes, turkey and rice. Stuff into peppers and place in a baking pan. Bake at 350° for 30 minutes. Top each pepper with about 1 tablespoon cheese. Return to oven for 3 minutes or until the cheese has melted. **Yield:** 6 servings.

Exchanges: 2 Meat, 2 Vegetable, 1 Starch

Nutritional Information

Serving Size: 1 stuffed pepper
Calories: 267
Sodium: 483 mg
Cholesterol: 51 mg
Carbohydrate: 29 gm
Protein: 21 gm
Fat: 10 gm

Lime Ginger Chicken

Patti Billet, Missoula, Montana

I find it very relaxing to spend a morning or afternoon in my kitchen trying new recipes. This recipe is one of my favorites—it won first prize in a statewide contest! The salsa is a fun and zippy addition.

1/3 cup fresh lime juice
   3 garlic cloves, minced
1/2 teaspoon ground ginger
1/2 teaspoon dried red pepper flakes
   4 boneless skinless chicken breast
      halves, cut into 1-inch strips
SALSA:
   2 cups diced fresh plum
      tomatoes
   1 cup diced green pepper
1/2 cup diced red onion
   1 tablespoon chopped fresh
      cilantro *or* parsley
   1 tablespoon olive *or* vegetable oil
   1 tablespoon fresh lime juice
   2 garlic cloves, minced

In a glass bowl, combine lime juice, garlic, ginger and red pepper. Add the chicken and toss lightly. Cover and refrigerate for 2-4 hours. Meanwhile, combine all salsa ingredients; cover and refrigerate until ready to serve. Drain chicken; discard marinade. Brown in a large nonstick skillet until no longer pink, about 10 minutes. Serve with salsa. **Yield:** 4 servings.

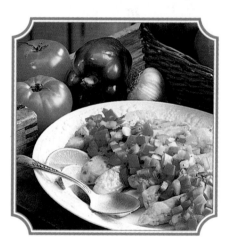

Exchanges: 3 Lean Meat, 3 Vegetable

Nutritional Information

Serving Size: 1/4 recipe
Calories: 250
Sodium: 80 mg
Cholesterol: 73 mg

Carbohydrate: 20 gm
Protein: 31 gm
Fat: 7 gm

Spicy Breaded Chicken

Polly Coumos, Mogadore, Ohio

(ALSO PICTURED ON FRONT COVER)

This is one of our family's favorite ways to make chicken.
The coating stays on, and the pan is easy to clean. We especially
like to pack this chicken cooked and chilled for picnics.

1/2 cup dry bread crumbs
1 tablespoon nonfat dry milk
   powder
1-1/2 teaspoons chili powder
1/4 teaspoon garlic powder
1/4 teaspoon dry mustard
1/4 cup skim milk
1 broiler-fryer chicken (3 pounds),
   cut into pieces and skin removed

In a plastic bag, mix bread crumbs, milk powder, chili powder, garlic powder and dry mustard; set aside. Pour milk into a shallow pan. Dip chicken pieces in milk, then place in bag and shake to coat. Place chicken, bone side down, in a 13-in. x 9-in. x 2-in. baking pan coated with non-stick cooking spray. Bake, uncovered, at 375° for 50-55 minutes or until juices run clear. **Yield:** 6 servings.

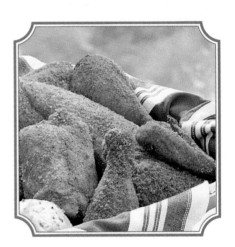

Exchanges: 4 Lean Meat, 1/2 Starch
Nutritional Information

Serving Size: 1/6 recipe
Calories: 233
Sodium: 154 mg
Cholesterol: 93 mg

Carbohydrate: 8 gm
Protein: 31 gm
Fat: 8 gm

Sunshine Chicken

Karen Gardiner, Eutaw, Alabama

Since it can be easily doubled and takes little time or effort to prepare, this recipe is great to serve for large groups. Even my husband, who usually doesn't enjoy cooking, likes to make this dish.

2 to 3 teaspoons curry powder
1/4 teaspoon pepper
6 boneless skinless chicken breast
    halves
1-1/2 cups orange juice
1 cup uncooked long grain rice
3/4 cup water
1 tablespoon brown sugar
1 teaspoon dry mustard
Chopped fresh parsley

Combine curry powder and pepper; rub over both sides of the chicken. In a skillet, combine orange juice, rice, water, brown sugar and mustard. Mix well. Top rice mixture with chicken pieces; bring to a boil. Cover and simmer 20-25 minutes. Remove from the heat and let stand, covered, until all liquid has absorbed, about 5 minutes. Sprinkle with parsley. **Yield:** 6 servings.

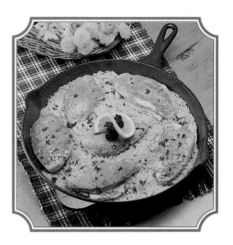

Exchanges: 2-1/2 Lean Meat, 2 Starch, 1 Fruit

Nutritional Information

Serving Size: 1/6 recipe
Calories: 304
Sodium: 66 mg
Cholesterol: 73 mg

Carbohydrate: 36 gm
Protein: 30 gm
Fat: 4 gm

Orange-Glazed Chicken

Diane Madonna, Brunswick, Ohio

A friend gave me this tasty recipe when I was living on a tight budget right after graduating from college. Today, it remains one of my favorite recipes. It's a sweet, tangy way to dress up a chicken breast.

1 tablespoon all-purpose flour
1/4 teaspoon pepper
1 boneless skinless chicken breast
  half
2 teaspoons vegetable oil
1/2 teaspoon orange marmalade
Dash ground nutmeg
1/2 cup orange juice
Hot cooked herbed rice, optional

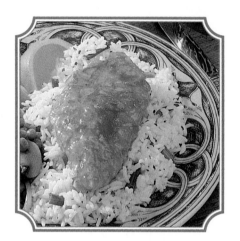

Combine flour and pepper; coat chicken breast. In a skillet, heat oil on medium; brown chicken. Spread marmalade on top of chicken; sprinkle with nutmeg. Add orange juice and simmer for 10-15 minutes or until the chicken juices run clear. Serve over rice if desired. **Yield:** 1 serving.

Exchanges: 4 Lean Meat, 1 Fat, 1 Fruit, 1/2 Starch

Nutritional Information

Serving Size: 1 recipe
Calories: 370
Sodium: 71 mg
Cholesterol: 83 mg

Carbohydrate: 23 gm
Protein: 31 gm
Fat: 17 gm
(Calculated without rice)

Grilled Lime Chicken

Lisa Dougherty, Vacaville, California

*My family is always delighted when I tell them
these grilled chicken breasts are on the menu. Everyone loves the
wonderful marinade...I relish the ease of preparation.*

**8 boneless skinless chicken breast
  halves**
1/2 cup lime juice
1/3 cup olive oil
4 green onions, chopped
4 garlic cloves, minced
**3 tablespoons chopped fresh dill,
  *divided***
1/4 teaspoon pepper

Pound chicken breasts to flatten. Combine lime juice, oil, onions, garlic, 2 tablespoons dill and pepper in a resealable plastic bag. Add chicken; seal and refrigerate 2-4 hours. Drain, discarding marinade. Grill chicken, uncovered, over medium-hot coals for 12-15 minutes, until tender and juices run clear. Turn after 6 minutes. Sprinkle with remaining dill before serving. **Yield:** 8 servings.

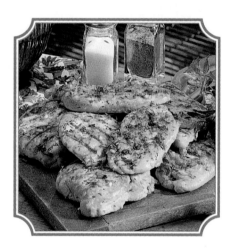

Exchanges: 3 Lean Meat, 1 Vegetable, 1 Fat
Nutritional Information
Serving Size: 1 chicken
breast half
Calories: 235
Sodium: 66 mg

Cholesterol: 73 mg
Carbohydrate: 3 gm
Protein: 27 gm
Fat: 12 gm

Light Chicken Kabobs

Margaret Balley, Coffeeville, Mississippi

Nothing captures the taste of summer like these flavorful kabobs sizzling on the grill. Best of all, they're easy to make ahead and grill in less than 30 minutes.

6 boneless skinless chicken breast halves
2 large green peppers, cut into 1-1/2-inch pieces
2 large onions, cut into 18 wedges
18 medium fresh mushrooms
1 bottle (8 ounces) low-fat Italian salad dressing
1/4 cup light soy sauce
1/4 cup Worcestershire sauce
2 tablespoons lemon juice

Cut each chicken breast half into three lengthwise strips. Place all ingredients in a glass bowl or large plastic bag; cover or seal. Stir or turn to coat. Refrigerate 4 hours or overnight, turning occasionally. Remove chicken and vegetables, reserving marinade. Thread alternately on 18 short skewers. Grill over medium-hot coals, turning and basting with marinade occasionally, for 12-15 minutes or until chicken juices run clear. **Yield:** 6 servings.

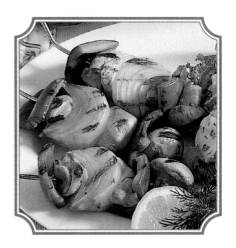

Exchanges: 3 Lean Meat, 2 Vegetable

Nutritional Information

Serving Size: 1/6 recipe
Calories: 210
Sodium: 673 mg
Cholesterol: 74 mg

Carbohydrate: 13 gm
Protein: 29 gm
Fat: 4 gm

Turkey Vegetable Skillet

June Formanek, Belle Plaine, Iowa

As everyone who raises a garden knows, zucchini grows overnight! I never let anything go to waste, so I try adding this hearty squash to every recipe I can. Out of all the recipes I've tried, this is my family's favorite.

1 pound ground turkey breast
1 small onion, chopped
1 garlic clove, minced
1 teaspoon vegetable oil
1 pound fresh tomatoes, chopped
1/4 pound zucchini, diced
1/4 cup chopped dill pickle
1 teaspoon dried basil
1/2 teaspoon pepper

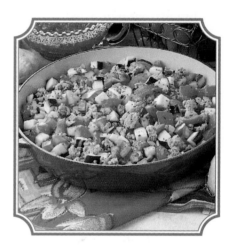

In a skillet, brown turkey, onion and garlic in oil. Add remaining ingredients. Simmer, uncovered, for 5-10 minutes or until the turkey is cooked and zucchini is tender. **Yield:** 6 servings.

Exchanges: 3 Lean Meat, 1 Vegetable
Nutritional Information
Serving Size: 1/6 recipe
Calories: 135
Sodium: 104 mg
Cholesterol: 47 mg

Carbohydrate: 5 gm
Protein: 21 gm
Fat: 3 gm

Lemon Chicken

Lori Schlecht, Wimbledon, North Dakota

*I originally tried this recipe because I love rice and chicken.
I made a few changes to suit my tastes and was pleased with
how it looks and the short time needed to prepare it.*

1 pound boneless skinless chicken
  breasts, cut into strips
1 medium onion, chopped
1 large carrot, thinly sliced
1 garlic clove, minced
2 tablespoons margarine
1 tablespoon cornstarch
1 can (14-1/2 ounces) low-sodium
  chicken broth
2 to 3 tablespoons fresh lemon
  juice
1 teaspoon grated lemon peel
1-1/2 cups uncooked instant rice
1 cup frozen chopped broccoli,
  thawed
1/4 cup minced fresh parsley

In a skillet, cook chicken, onion, carrot and garlic in margarine until chicken is lightly browned, about 5 minutes. In a bowl, combine the cornstarch and broth; stir in lemon juice, peel and rice. Add to skillet and bring to a boil. Reduce heat; add broccoli and parsley. Cover and simmer 5-10 minutes or until rice is tender. **Yield:** 4 servings.

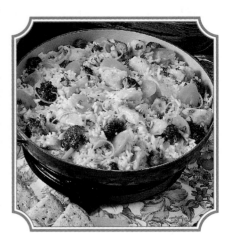

Exchanges: 3 Lean Meat, 2 Starch, 1 Vegetable

Nutritional Information

Serving Size: 1/4 recipe
Calories: 367
Sodium: 132 mg
Cholesterol: 73 mg

Carbohydrate: 39 gm
Protein: 31 gm
Fat: 9 gm

Turkey Curry

Martha Balser, Cincinnati, Ohio

I'm always looking for new and interesting ways to use leftover turkey—especially around the holidays. This is a zesty entree you can make as spicy as you like by varying the amount of curry powder.

1 cup sliced celery
1/2 cup sliced carrots
1 cup skim milk, *divided*
2 tablespoons cornstarch
3/4 cup low-sodium chicken broth
2 tablespoons dried minced onion
1/2 teaspoon garlic powder
1 to 4 teaspoons curry powder
2 cups diced cooked turkey breast
Hot cooked rice, optional

Lightly coat a skillet with nonstick cooking spray; saute celery and carrots until tender. In a bowl, mix 1/4 cup milk and cornstarch until smooth. Add broth and remaining milk; mix until smooth. Pour over vegetables in skillet. Add onion, garlic powder and curry powder. Cook and stir over medium heat for 4-5 minutes or until mixture thickens and bubbles. Add turkey; cook and stir until heated through. Serve over rice if desired. **Yield:** 4 servings.

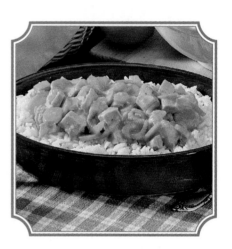

Exchanges: 2-1/2 Lean Meat, 1 Vegetable, 1/2 Starch, 1/2 Skim Milk

Nutritional Information

Serving Size: 1 cup
Calories: 232
Sodium: 206 mg
Cholesterol: 37 mg

Carbohydrate: 15 gm
Protein: 29 gm
Fat: 6 gm
(Calculated without rice)

Oatmeal Baked Chicken

Ena Quiggle, Goodhue, Minnesota

This recipe proves you can have fried chicken without a lot of fuss. The chili powder and cumin add a subtle spiciness that appeals to everyone.

1-1/2 cups quick-cooking oats
1 tablespoon paprika
1 tablespoon chili powder
3/4 teaspoon garlic powder
1/2 teaspoon ground cumin
1/4 teaspoon pepper
1 broiler-fryer chicken (4 pounds), cut up
1/2 cup skim milk
2 tablespoons margarine, melted

Coat a 13-in. x 9-in. x 2-in. baking dish with nonstick cooking spray; set aside. In a shallow bowl or large resealable plastic bag, combine oats, paprika, chili powder, garlic powder, cumin and pepper. Dip chicken in milk, then coat with oat mixture. Place in prepared baking dish. Drizzle with margarine. Bake, uncovered, at 375° for 45-50 minutes or until juices run clear. **Yield:** 4 servings.

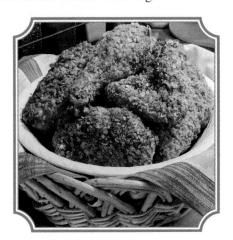

Exchanges: 3 Lean Meat, 1–1/2 Starch, 1 Fat

Nutritional Information

Serving Size: 1/4 recipe
Calories: 316
Sodium: 146 mg
Cholesterol: 62 mg

Carbohydrate: 24 gm
Protein: 28 gm
Fat: 12 gm

Orange Chicken

Irma Collison, Pigeon, Michigan

This chicken has a fresh and fruity citrus flavor that is sure to satisfy your family. I've been asked to make this more times than I can remember!

1 broiler-fryer chicken (3-1/2 to 4 pounds), cut up and skin removed
1 can (6 ounces) frozen orange juice concentrate, thawed
2 teaspoons lemon juice
1 teaspoon low-sodium chicken bouillon granules
1 teaspoon ground savory
1/2 teaspoon ground sage

Place chicken pieces in a 13-in. x 9-in. x 2-in. baking dish coated with nonstick cooking spray. Combine orange juice, lemon juice, bouillon, savory and sage; pour over chicken. Bake, uncovered, at 350° for 60-70 minutes or until juices run clear, basting occasionally. **Yield:** 4 servings.

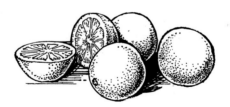

Exchanges: 2-1/2 Lean Meat, 2 Fruit

Nutritional Information

Serving Size: 1/4 recipe
Calories: 253
Sodium: 74 mg
Cholesterol: 62 mg

Carbohydrate: 30 gm
Protein: 24 gm
Fat: 4 gm

Low-Fat Chicken Divan

Debbie Wheeler, Nampa, Idaho

*This is a nutritious dish that doesn't skimp on taste.
Get ready for rave reviews when you serve this creamy casserole.*

1-1/4 pounds chopped fresh broccoli, cooked
3 cups cubed cooked chicken
1 can (10-3/4 ounces) condensed low-fat cream of chicken soup, undiluted
1 cup low-sodium chicken broth
1 cup fat-free mayonnaise
2 tablespoons fresh lemon juice
1/2 teaspoon pepper
1/4 teaspoon garlic powder
3/4 cup shredded low-fat cheddar cheese

Spray a 13-in. x 9-in. x 2-in. baking pan with nonstick cooking spray. Arrange the broccoli in the pan; cover with chicken. Combine the next six ingredients; pour over the chicken. Sprinkle with cheese. Cover and bake at 350° for 30 minutes. Uncover; bake 5-10 minutes or until bubbly. **Yield:** 6 servings.

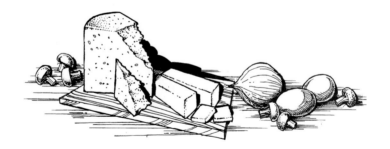

Exchanges: 2 Lean Meat, 1 Starch, 1 Vegetable
Nutritional Information

Serving Size: 1/6 recipe
Calories: 201
Sodium: 501 mg
Cholesterol: 63 mg

Carbohydrate: 17 gm
Protein: 20 gm
Fat: 5 gm

Pork

Whether it's prepared in a sizzling
skillet supper, one-dish oven meal or
cookout classic, versatile pork always pleases.

Orange Pork Chops

Elaine Fenton, Prescott, Arizona

I'm constantly on the lookout for ways to "spice up" a standard dish. When I fixed these pork chops for the first time, my husband—who has a hearty appetite for down-home cooking—commented, "You can make this anytime!"

6 pork loin chops (1/2 inch thick)
1 tablespoon cooking oil
3/4 cup water
1/2 teaspoon paprika
1/2 teaspoon pepper
1 medium orange
1/2 cup sugar
1 tablespoon cornstarch
1/2 teaspoon ground cinnamon
12 whole cloves
1 cup fresh orange juice

In a large skillet, brown chops in oil on both sides. Add water, paprika and pepper; bring to a boil. Reduce heat to low; cover and simmer about 35 minutes, turning once. Meanwhile, grate peel from the stem end of the orange, then cut six slices from the other end. Set aside. In a saucepan over medium-high, combine 1 tablespoon peel, sugar, cornstarch, cinnamon and cloves. Stir in juice. Cook and stir until thickened. Add orange slices; cover and remove from the heat. To serve, top chops with sauce and orange slices. **Yield:** 6 servings.

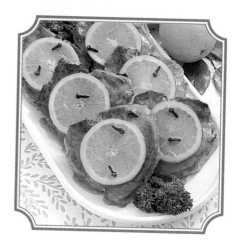

Exchanges: 2-1/2 Meat, 1/2 Fruit
Nutritional Information
Serving Size: 1 pork chop
Calories: 208
Sodium: 30 mg
Cholesterol: 50 mg

Carbohydrate: 9 gm
Protein: 18 gm
Fat: 11 gm

Sweet-and-Sour Pork

Arly Schnabel, Ellendale, North Dakota

This is an easy recipe—and it comes in mighty handy at the end of a busy workday! I enjoy collecting cookbooks and am always looking for new ideas.

1 can (20 ounces) pineapple
   chunks in natural juices,
   liquid drained and reserved
1/2 cup water
1 tablespoon cornstarch
3 tablespoons light soy sauce
1 teaspoon vinegar
1/4 teaspoon crushed red pepper
   flakes
2 tablespoons cooking oil
1 pound boneless pork loin, cut
   into thin strips
2 garlic cloves, minced
1 teaspoon ground ginger
2 medium carrots, thinly sliced
1 medium onion, cut into wedges
1 green *or* sweet red pepper,
   thinly sliced
2 cups snow peas, trimmed
Hot cooked rice, optional

Combine 3 tablespoons reserved pineapple juice with water, cornstarch, soy sauce, vinegar and red pepper flakes. Set aside. In a skillet or wok, heat oil on high. Stir-fry pork until no longer pink. Add garlic and ginger; cook 1 minute. Add carrots and onion; continue to stir-fry until tender, about 3 minutes. Add green pepper, peas, pineapple and soy sauce mixture that has been stirred. Cook until sauce thickens. Serve over rice if desired. **Yield:** 4 servings.

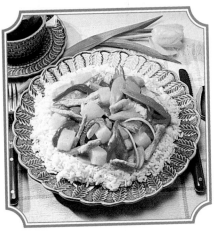

Exchanges: 2 Meat, 1-1/2 Fruit, 1-1/2 Vegetable, 1 Fat

Nutritional Information

Serving Size: 1/4 recipe
Calories: 335
Sodium: 232 mg
Cholesterol: 60 mg

Carbohydrate: 28 gm
Protein: 21 gm
Fat: 16 gm
(Calculated without rice)

Chalupa (Mexican Stew)

Anne Fatout, Phoenix, Arizona

We've lived in Arizona for 40 years, so Mexican cooking has become the same as "Arizona cooking" for us. Nothing tastes better than this stew!

1 pound dry pinto beans
1 pork roast (3 pounds), trimmed
4 to 5 garlic cloves, minced
2 tablespoons chili powder
1 to 1-1/2 teaspoons ground cumin
1 teaspoon dried oregano
2 cans (4 ounces *each*) chopped
   green chilies
Pepper to taste
5 carrots, peeled and sliced
4 celery ribs, sliced
1 can (14-1/2 ounces) tomatoes
   with liquid, cut up
3 small zucchini, sliced
Flour tortillas, warmed, optional

Soak beans overnight; drain. Place in a large Dutch oven or kettle. Add the next seven ingredients. Cover with water and cook, covered, over low heat 3-4 hours or until meat and beans are tender. Cool slightly; remove meat from bones. Cut or shred meat into bite-size pieces; return to kettle. Add carrots, celery and tomatoes; cover and cook until vegetables are tender. Add zucchini during the last 10 minutes. Serve with warmed tortillas if desired. **Yield:** 16 servings.

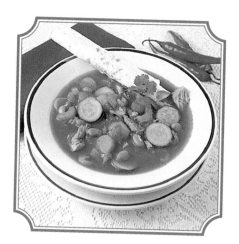

Exchanges: 1-1/2 Starch, 1-1/2 Meat, 1 Vegetable

Nutritional Information

Serving Size: 1 cup
Calories: 253
Sodium: 160 mg
Cholesterol: 41 mg

Carbohydrate: 26 gm
Protein: 22 gm
Fat: 7 gm
(Calculated without tortillas)

Spiedis

Gertrude Skinner, Binghamton, New York

This is our favorite cookout dish. The recipe originated here in my hometown in the 1930's. Our meat preference for spiedis is venison, but we use others when it's not available.

1 cup vegetable oil
2/3 cup cider vinegar
2 tablespoons Worcestershire
   sauce
1/2 medium onion, finely chopped
1/2 teaspoon sugar
1/2 teaspoon dried basil
1/2 teaspoon dried marjoram
1/2 teaspoon dried rosemary
2-1/2 pounds boneless lean pork, beef,
   lamb, venison, chicken *or*
   turkey, cut into 1-1/2- to 2-inch
   cubes
Rolls *or* bread of your choice

In a glass dish, combine first eight ingredients. Add meat and toss to coat. Cover and refrigerate for 24 hours, stirring occasionally. When ready to cook, thread meat on metal skewers and grill over hot coals until meat reaches desired doneness, about 10-15 minutes. Remove meat from skewers and serve on rolls or bread. **Yield:** 8 servings.

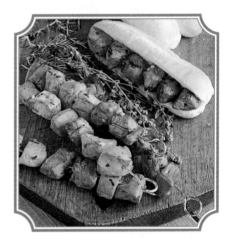

Exchanges: 3 Lean Meat, 1 Fat

Nutritional Information

Serving Size: 1/8 recipe
Calories: 205
Sodium: 104 mg
Cholesterol: 42 mg

Carbohydrate: 1 gm
Protein: 22 gm
Fat: 12 gm
(Calculated without bread)

One-Dish Pork Chop Dinner

Pat Waymire, Yellow Springs, Ohio

This is a delicious meaty main dish. The apple juice gives the pork a wonderful flavor, and the cabbage taste isn't too strong.

8 pork chops (1/2 inch thick)
1/3 cup all-purpose flour
1/4 cup margarine
Pepper to taste
    2 cups apple juice, *divided*
    2 pounds small red potatoes
    1 pound *or* **1 jar (16 ounces)**
    small whole onions, drained
    1 pound carrots, cut into 3-inch
    pieces
    6 to 8 cups shredded cabbage

Coat pork chops in flour; reserve excess flour. In a large Dutch oven, melt margarine over medium-high heat. Brown chops on both sides. Season with pepper. Remove and set aside. Stir reserved flour into pan; cook and stir until a paste forms. Gradually whisk in 1-1/2 cups apple juice; blend until smooth. Return chops to Dutch oven; cover and bake at 350° for 30 minutes. Add potatoes, onions, carrots and remaining apple juice. Cover and bake 30 minutes longer. Top with cabbage; cover and bake for 1 to 1-1/2 hours or until the pork chops are tender, basting occasionally. **Yield:** 8 servings.

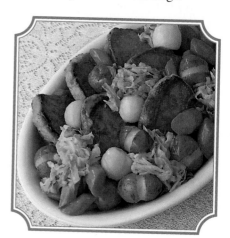

Exchanges: 2-1/2 Fat, 2 Meat, 2 Starch, 2 Vegetable
Nutritional Information
Serving Size: 1/8 recipe
Calories: 464
Sodium: 333 mg
Cholesterol: 56 mg
Carbohydrate: 43 gm
Protein: 19 gm
Fat: 24 gm

Orange Ham Kabobs

DeAnn Alleva, Charlotte, North Carolina

When I want to liven up leftover ham, I often make this main meal. It's a new and interesting way to prepare kabobs, and they're always a hit!

1-1/2 pounds fully cooked ham, cut into 24 cubes (1-inch pieces)
2 medium oranges, peeled and cut into eighths
1 large green pepper, cut into 16 pieces
1 large sweet red pepper, cut into 16 pieces
1/2 cup orange juice
2 tablespoons tomato paste
1/4 teaspoon ground ginger

On eight metal skewers, alternately thread three ham cubes, two orange pieces, two green pepper pieces and two red pepper pieces. Place on a broiler pan with rack; broil 4-5 in. from the heat for 8 minutes, turning occasionally. In a small bowl, combine the orange juice, tomato paste and ginger; mix well. Brush half over kabobs; broil 2-3 minutes. Turn kabobs and brush with the remaining sauce; broil 2 minutes more or until the vegetables are tender. **Yield:** 8 servings.

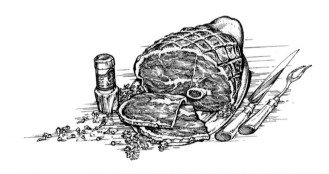

Exchanges: 3 Lean Meat
Nutritional Information

Serving Size: 1 kabob
Calories: 150
Sodium: 1,248 mg
Cholesterol: 40 mg

Carbohydrate: 10 gm
Protein: 17 gm
Fat: 5 gm

Herbed Pork Roast

Dianne Bettin, Truman, Minnesota

*This recipe deliciously proves that pork roasts don't have to be
loaded with fat and calories to be satisfying. Even folks
not on restricted diets will find this roast appealing.*

3 tablespoons finely chopped fresh
  parsley, *divided*
2 teaspoons paprika
2 teaspoons dried basil
1 teaspoon pepper
1 teaspoon garlic powder
1 teaspoon dried oregano
1/2 teaspoon crushed fennel seed
1/2 teaspoon dried thyme
1 boneless extra-lean pork roast
  (about 2 pounds)

Combine half of the parsley with the
herbs and seasonings. Rub over roast.
Place in a shallow pan; cover with remaining parsley. Roast, uncovered, at
325° for 35 minutes *per pound* or until
the internal temperature reaches 160°-
170°. **Yield:** 6 servings.

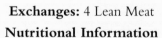

Exchanges: 4 Lean Meat

Nutritional Information

Serving Size: 1/6 recipe
Calories: 239
Sodium: 86 mg
Cholesterol: 98 mg

Carbohydrate: 98 gm
Protein: 32 gm
Fat: 11 gm

Pork and Winter Squash Stew

Evelyn Plyler, Apple Valley, California

*Here in the high desert area of California, we do get snow.
So this stew's especially popular in winter!*

**2 pounds lean boneless pork, cut
   into 1-inch cubes
2 tablespoons cooking oil,** *divided*
**2 cups chopped onion
2 garlic cloves, minced
3 cups sliced fresh mushrooms
2-1/2 cups diagonally sliced carrots
2 cans (14-1/2 ounces** *each***)
   Italian stewed tomatoes
2 teaspoons dried thyme
1/2 teaspoon pepper
4 cups cubed peeled butternut
   squash
Hot cooked noodles, optional**

In a 4-qt. Dutch oven, brown pork in 1 tablespoon of oil. Remove from pan; drain
and set aside. Heat remaining oil in the
same pan over medium heat. Saute onion
and garlic for 3 minutes. Return pork to
pan. Add mushrooms, carrots, tomatoes,
thyme and pepper; bring to a boil. Reduce
heat; cover and simmer for 1 hour. Add
squash; simmer, uncovered, for 30 minutes or until meat and vegetables are tender. Serve over noodles if desired. **Yield:**
8 servings.

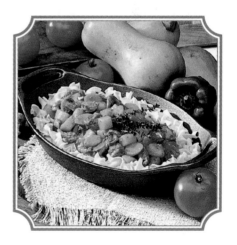

Exchanges: 2 Meat, 2 Vegetable, 1 Starch, 1 Fat
Nutritional Information
Serving Size: 1/8 recipe
Calories: 298
Sodium: 393 mg
Cholesterol: 60 mg

Carbohydrate: 26 gm
Protein: 22 gm
Fat: 14 gm
(Calculated without noodles)

Spicy Pork Tenderloin

Diana Steger, Prospect, Kentucky

*A friend shared this recipe for marvelously flavorful pork years ago.
It really sparks up a barbecue and has been popular whenever I've served it.
I guarantee you'll get many requests for the recipe.*

**1 to 3 tablespoons chili powder
1 teaspoon salt
1/4 teaspoon ground ginger
1/4 teaspoon ground thyme
1/4 teaspoon pepper
2 pork tenderloins (about
1 pound *each*)**

Combine the first five ingredients; rub over tenderloins. Cover and refrigerate for 2-4 hours. Grill over hot coals for 15 minutes per side or until juices run clear or the internal temperature reaches 160°. **Yield:** 8 servings.

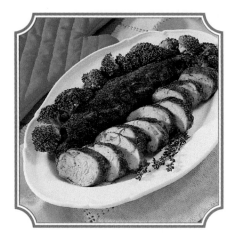

Exchanges: 3-1/2 Lean Meat

Nutritional Information

Serving Size: 1/8 recipe
Calories: 173
Sodium: 328 mg
Cholesterol: 93 mg

Carbohydrate: 1 gm
Protein: 29 gm
Fat: 5 gm

Asparagus Ham Rolls

Laurie Timm, Minneiska, Minnesota

I love this delicious recipe because it includes three of my favorite locally produced foods—ham, asparagus and cheese. Prepared with leftover ham and fresh asparagus, these rolls make an excellent meal.

2 tablespoons margarine
1/4 cup all-purpose flour
2 cups skim milk
1/2 cup shredded cheddar cheese
1/4 teaspoon white pepper
24 fresh *or* frozen asparagus
stalks
8 thin slices fully cooked ham
(about 1/2 pound)
1/4 cup soft bread crumbs

In a saucepan, melt margarine; stir in flour and cook until thick. Gradually stir in milk and cook until bubbly and thickened. Stir in cheese and pepper. Remove from the heat. Place three asparagus stalks on each ham slice. Roll up; secure with toothpicks if necessary. Place in an ungreased 13-in. x 9-in. x 2-in. baking pan; cover with cheese sauce. Sprinkle with crumbs. Bake, uncovered, at 375° for 20 minutes. **Yield:** 8 servings.

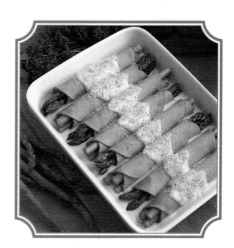

Exchanges: 1 Meat, 1 Vegetable, 1/2 Starch

Nutritional Information

Serving Size: 1 roll-up
Calories: 125
Sodium: 418 mg
Cholesterol: 19 mg

Carbohydrate: 11 gm
Protein: 11 gm
Fat: 7 gm

Green Chili Pork Stew

Pat Henderson, Deer Park, Texas

Green chilies are a big favorite here in the Southwest—my family likes anything with them in it. My husband is used to me springing at least one new recipe on him each week. He's always brave!

2 pounds lean boneless pork, cut into 1-1/2-inch cubes
1 tablespoon cooking oil
4 cups low-sodium chicken broth, *divided*
3 cans (11 ounces *each*) whole kernel corn, drained
2 celery ribs, diced
2 medium potatoes, peeled and diced
2 medium tomatoes, diced
3 cans (4 ounces *each*) chopped green chilies
2 teaspoons ground cumin
1 teaspoon dried oregano
3 tablespoons all-purpose flour

In a 5-qt. Dutch oven over medium-high heat, brown pork in oil. Add 3-1/2 cups broth, corn, celery, potatoes, tomatoes, chilies, cumin and oregano; bring to a boil.

Reduce heat; cover and simmer for 1 hour or until meat and vegetables are tender. Combine flour and remaining broth; stir into stew. Bring to a boil; cook, stirring constantly, until thickened. **Yield:** 8 servings.

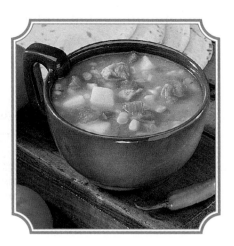

Exchanges: 2 Meat, 2 Vegetable, 1 Starch, 1 Fat

Nutritional Information

Serving Size: 1/8 recipe
Calories: 306
Sodium: 466 mg
Cholesterol: 60 mg

Carbohydrate: 27 gm
Protein: 23 gm
Fat: 12 gm

Skillet Pork Chops with Zucchini

Diane Banaszak, West Bend, Wisconsin

We're always blessed with plenty of zucchini from our garden in summer, so I try lots of different zucchini recipes. This is one of my family's favorites.

3 tablespoons all-purpose flour
5 tablespoons grated Parmesan
  cheese, *divided*
1-1/2 teaspoons salt
  1/2 teaspoon dill weed
  1/4 teaspoon pepper
  6 pork chops (about 3/4 inch
    thick)
  1 tablespoon cooking oil
  2 medium onions, sliced
  1/3 cup water
  3 medium zucchini (about
    1 pound), sliced
  1/2 teaspoon paprika

In a large plastic bag, combine flour, 2 tablespoons Parmesan cheese, salt, dill and pepper. Place pork chops in bag and shake to coat; shake off excess flour and reserve. Heat oil in a large skillet over medium-high; brown pork chops on both sides. Reduce heat. Place onion slices on chops. Add water to skillet; cover and simmer for 15 minutes. Place zucchini slices over the onion. Mix remaining Parmesan cheese with reserved flour mixture; sprinkle over zucchini. Sprinkle paprika on top. Cover and simmer for 25 minutes or until pork chops are tender. **Yield:** 6 servings.

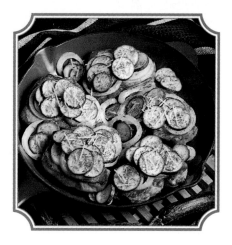

Exchanges: 3 Meat, 1-1/2 Vegetable
Nutritional Information
Serving Size: 1/6 recipe
Calories: 279
Sodium: 638 mg
Cholesterol: 78 mg

Carbohydrate: 9 gm
Protein: 27 gm
Fat: 15 gm

Pork Stroganoff

Janice Mitchell, Aurora, Colorado

I do most of my cooking from scratch, and this hearty dish is no exception. It features tender chunks of pork in a deliciously creamy sauce.

1-1/2 pounds pork stew meat, cut into 1-1/2-inch cubes
1-1/2 cups water, *divided*
1 teaspoon low-sodium instant chicken bouillon granules
2 teaspoons paprika
1 cup chopped onion
1 garlic clove, minced
1 tablespoon cornstarch
3/4 cup light sour cream
2 tablespoons snipped fresh parsley

In a large saucepan coated with nonstick cooking spray, brown the pork; drain. Remove and set aside. In the same saucepan, bring 1-1/4 cups water, bouillon and paprika to a boil. Add pork, onion and garlic; reduce heat. Cover and simmer for 45 minutes or until meat is tender. Combine the cornstarch and remaining water; gradually add to meat mixture, stirring constantly. Bring to a boil; cook and stir for 2 minutes or until thickened. Remove from the heat. Stir in sour cream and parsley. **Yield:** 6 servings.

Exchanges: 4 Lean Meat, 1/2 Starch
Nutritional Information

Serving Size: 1/6 recipe
Calories: 251
Sodium: 99 mg
Cholesterol: 76 mg

Carbohydrate: 8 gm
Protein: 30 gm
Fat: 12 gm

Grilled Apricot Ham

Mary Ann Kosmas, Minneapolis, Minnesota

Here in Minnesota, summers never seem to last long enough! So we take advantage of warm weather and head to the outdoors for good old-fashioned cookouts. This grilled ham steak is quick and easy for weekday dinners, yet impressive enough for special-occasion meals.

1/4 cup all-fruit apricot spread
2 teaspoons Dijon mustard
2 teaspoons cider vinegar
1 ham steak (about 1 pound)

In a small bowl, combine apricot spread, mustard and vinegar. Grill ham steak over hot coals, brushing occasionally with sauce, until browned on both sides, about 8-10 minutes. **Yield:** 4 servings.

SIMPLE SOLUTION. Avoid the sticky situation of food getting stuck on your grill. Spray a *cold* grill rack—away from open flames—with nonstick cooking spray before beginning your barbecue.

Exchanges: 3 Lean Meat, 1 Fruit
Nutritional Information

Serving Size: 1/4 recipe
Calories: 205
Sodium: 1,654 mg
Cholesterol: 53 mg

Carbohydrate: 15 gm
Protein: 22 gm
Fat: 5 gm

Pork Tenderloin Diane

Janie Thorpe, Tullahoma, Tennessee

We have pork at least once a week, and this is one dish we especially enjoy. Moist tender pork "medallions" are served up in a savory sauce for a combination that's irresistible.

1 pork tenderloin (about 1 pound)
1 tablespoon lemon-pepper seasoning
2 tablespoons margarine
2 tablespoons lemon juice
1 tablespoon Worcestershire sauce
1 teaspoon Dijon mustard
1 tablespoon minced fresh parsley

Cut tenderloin into eight pieces; place each piece between two pieces of plastic wrap or waxed paper and flatten to 1/2-in. thickness. Sprinkle with lemon pepper. Melt margarine in a large skillet over medium heat; cook pork for 3-4 minutes on each side or until no longer pink and juices run clear. Remove to a serving platter and keep warm. To the pan juices, add lemon juice, Worcestershire sauce and mustard; heat through, stirring occasionally. Pour over the pork and sprinkle with parsley. Serve immediately. **Yield:** 4 servings.

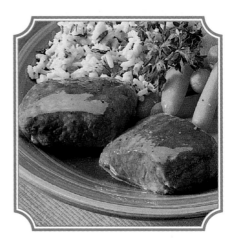

Exchanges: 3 Meat

Nutritional Information

Serving Size: 2 pork medallions
Calories: 214
Sodium: 491 mg
Cholesterol: 6 mg

Carbohydrate: 1 gm
Protein: 18 gm
Fat: 14 gm

Pork Chow Mein

Helen Carpenter, Marble Falls, Texas

I give all the credit for my love of cooking and baking to my mother, grandmother and mother-in-law. That trio inspired delicious dishes like this hearty skillet dinner. When we get a taste for stir-fry, this dish really hits the spot.

1 pound boneless pork loin
2 garlic cloves, minced
4 tablespoons light soy sauce,
  divided
1 cup low-sodium chicken broth
2 tablespoons cornstarch
1/2 to 1 teaspoon ground ginger
1 tablespoon cooking oil
1 cup thinly sliced carrots
1 cup thinly sliced celery
1 cup chopped onion
1 cup coarsely chopped cabbage
1 cup coarsely chopped fresh
  spinach
Hot cooked rice, optional

Cut pork into 4-in. x 1/2-in. x 1/4-in. strips; place in a bowl. Add garlic and 2 tablespoons soy sauce. Cover and refrigerate 2-4 hours. Meanwhile, combine broth, cornstarch, ginger and remaining soy sauce; mix well and set aside. Heat oil in a large skillet or wok on high; stir-fry pork until no longer pink. Remove and keep warm. Add carrots and celery; stir-fry 3-4 minutes. Add onion, cabbage and spinach; stir-fry 2-3 minutes. Stir broth mixture and add to skillet along with pork. Cook and stir until broth thickens, about 3-4 minutes. Serve over rice if desired. **Yield:** 6 servings.

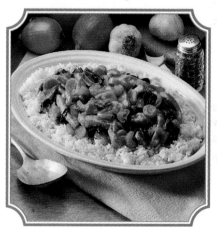

Exchanges: 2 Meat, 1 Vegetable

Nutritional Information

Serving Size: 1/6 recipe
Calories: 173
Sodium: 419 mg
Cholesterol: 40 mg

Carbohydrate: 11 gm
Protein: 14 gm
Fat: 8 gm
(Calculated without rice)

Marinated Pork Kabobs

Bobbie Jo Devany, Fernly, Nevada

This recipe was originally for lamb, but I adapted it to pork and adjusted the spices. After tasting these flavorful kabobs, my husband became an instant fan of this recipe. It's always requested when the grill comes out for the season.

2 cups plain low-fat yogurt
2 tablespoons lemon juice
4 garlic cloves, minced
1/2 teaspoon ground cumin
1/4 teaspoon ground coriander
2 pounds pork tenderloin, cut
    into 1-1/2-inch cubes
8 small white onions, halved
8 cherry tomatoes
1 medium sweet red pepper,
    cut into 1-1/2-inch pieces
1 medium green pepper, cut
    into 1-1/2-inch pieces

In a medium glass bowl, combine yogurt, lemon juice, garlic, cumin and coriander; mix well. Add pork; cover and refrigerate for 6 hours or overnight. Alternate pork, onions, tomatoes and peppers on eight skewers. Grill over medium coals for about 30-35 minutes or until meat reaches desired doneness. **Yield:** 8 servings.

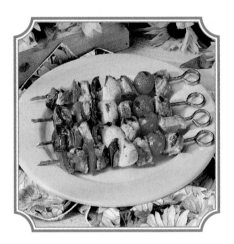

Exchanges: 4 Lean Meat, 2 Vegetable, 1/2 Fat

Nutritional Information

Serving Size: 1 kabob
Calories: 299
Sodium: 87 mg
Cholesterol: 94 mg

Carbohydrate: 8 gm
Protein: 31 gm
Fat: 7 gm

Barbecued Pork Sandwiches

Thelma Waggoner, Hopkinsville, Kentucky

These delicious sandwiches taste even better if the pork is prepared a day ahead for the flavors to blend. Growing up, we welcomed Mother's pork sandwiches for any occasion, but especially for our birthday celebration.

1 pork shoulder roast (about 5 pounds), trimmed and cut into 1-inch cubes
2 medium onions, coarsely chopped
2 tablespoons chili powder
1-1/2 cups water
1 cup ketchup
1/4 cup vinegar
Bread *or* rolls of your choice

In a Dutch oven, combine meat, onions, chili powder, water, ketchup and vinegar. Cover and simmer for 4 hours or until the meat falls apart easily. Skim off the excess fat. With a slotted spoon, remove meat, reserving cooking liquid. Shred the meat with two forks. Return to the cooking liquid and heat through. Serve on bread or rolls. **Yield:** 16 servings.

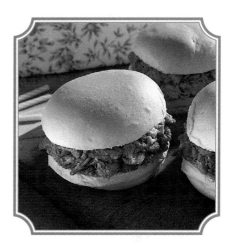

Exchanges: 3 Lean Meat, 1 Vegetable
Nutritional Information

Serving Size: 1/2 cup
Calories: 202
Sodium: 219 mg
Cholesterol: 84 mg

Carbohydrate: 4 gm
Protein: 24 gm
Fat: 9 gm
(Calculated without bread)

Grilled Pork Tenderloin

Lillian Owens, New Castle, Kentucky

Who says recipes have to be fancy in order to be flavorful?
We have a lot of cookouts around our house, and this pork tenderloin
is a favorite of ours when we're eating outdoors. It's simple to prepare...
and simply delicious. Everyone who tries it requests the recipe.

2 pork tenderloins (about 1 pound
**   *each*)**
1 bottle (8 ounces) low-fat Italian
**   salad dressing**

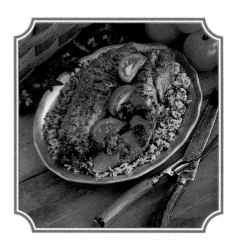

Place tenderloins in a glass bowl. Pour dressing over. Cover and refrigerate for 6-8 hours or overnight. Grill over hot coals for 15-20 minutes or until juices run clear or the internal temperature reaches 160°. Slice and serve immediately. **Yield:** 6 servings.

Exchanges: 3-1/2 Lean Meat, 1/2 Fat
Nutritional Information

Serving Size: 1/6 recipe
Calories: 230
Sodium: 217 mg
Cholesterol: 74 mg

Carbohydrate: trace
Protein: 24 gm
Fat: 14 gm

New York-Style Spiedis

Beatrice Riddell, Chenango Bridge, New York

Spiedi–Fest is held in a nearby town each summer and thousands of people attend. This recipe is my own, but there are many variations in our area. I hope you enjoy it!

4 pounds pork tenderloin, cut into 1-inch cubes
2 cups tomato juice
2 large onions, finely chopped
4 to 5 garlic cloves, minced
2 tablespoons Worcestershire sauce
2 teaspoons chopped fresh basil *or* **1 teaspoon dried basil**
Pepper to taste
Bread of your choice

In a large glass bowl, combine the first seven ingredients. Cover and refrigerate overnight. Drain, discarding marinade. Thread pork on small skewers, using five per skewer; grill or broil for 15-20 minutes, turning occasionally, until the meat is no longer pink and pulls away easily from the skewers. To serve, wrap a slice of bread around meat and pull off skewer. **Yield:** 12 servings.

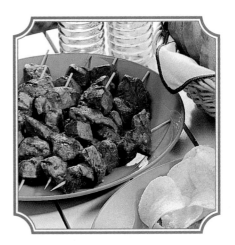

Exchanges: 4 Lean Meat

Nutritional Information

Serving Size: 1/12 recipe
Calories: 214
Sodium: 152 mg
Cholesterol: 77 mg

Carbohydrate: 1 gm
Protein: 24 gm
Fat: 12 gm
(Calculated without bread)

Savory Pork Stew

Jodi Bierschenk, Newhall, Iowa

Stews are one of my favorite foods. They can be put together to simmer, leaving me time to get things done around the house. I know you'll appreciate the convenience of this one-dish meal.

1 pound lean boneless pork, cut into 1-inch cubes
1 cup chopped onion
1 teaspoon dried basil
1/2 teaspoon dried rosemary, crushed
1/4 teaspoon pepper
1/2 cup water
1 can (16 ounces) tomato sauce
2 cups sliced carrots
1 green pepper, chopped
1/2 pound fresh mushrooms, sliced

Place pork in a Dutch oven that has been sprayed with nonstick cooking spray. Cook over medium heat until browned. Add onion, seasonings, water and tomato sauce; bring to a boil. Reduce heat; cover and simmer 1 hour or until meat is tender. Stir in remaining ingredients. Cover and simmer until the vegetables are tender, about 30 minutes. **Yield:** 5 servings.

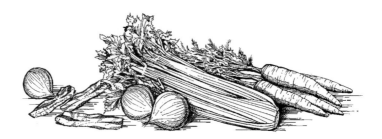

Exchanges: 3 Vegetable, 2 Lean Meat
Nutritional Information

Serving Size: 1/5 recipe
Calories: 201
Sodium: 644 mg
Cholesterol: 48 mg

Carbohydrate: 15 gm
Protein: 18 gm
Fat: 7 gm

Fish & Seafood

Fishing for flavorful food in a flash?
Folks will fall for these fabulous dishes...
hook, line and sinker!

Baked Lemon Haddock

Jean Ann Perkins, Newburyport, Maryland

Fish products are abundant here on the East Coast, so I'm always in search of new and fun ways to prepare it. Our family never tires of this simply superb baked fish. As a matter of fact, it's my husband's favorite.

2 pounds haddock fillets
1 cup seasoned dry bread crumbs
1/4 cup margarine, melted
2 tablespoons dried parsley flakes
2 teaspoons grated lemon peel
1/2 teaspoon garlic powder

Cut fish into serving-size pieces. Place in an 11-in. x 7-in. x 2-in. baking dish coated with nonstick cooking spray. Combine remaining ingredients; sprinkle over fish. Bake at 350° for 25 minutes or until fish flakes easily with a fork. **Yield:** 6 servings.

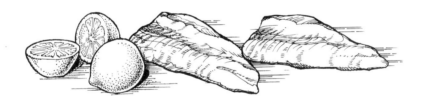

Exchanges: 3 Lean Meat, 1 Starch
Nutritional Information

Serving Size: 1/6 recipe
Calories: 239
Sodium: 650 mg
Cholesterol: 67 mg

Carbohydrate: 15 gm
Protein: 25 gm
Fat: 9 gm

Sole in Herbed Butter

Marilyn Paradis, Woodburn, Oregon

I often rely on seafood recipes for quick meals. This flavorful fish is easy to make and is ready in just a few minutes. I know your family will request this often throughout the year!

4 tablespoons light margarine, softened
1 teaspoon dill weed
1/2 teaspoon onion powder
1/2 teaspoon garlic powder
1/4 teaspoon white pepper
2 pounds sole fillets

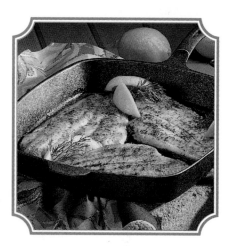

In a bowl, mix margarine, dill, onion powder, garlic powder and pepper. Transfer to a skillet; heat on medium until melted. Add the sole and saute for several minutes on each side or until it flakes easily with a fork. **Yield:** 6 servings.

Exchanges: 4-1/2 Lean Meat, 1/2 Fat

Nutritional Information

Serving Size: 1/6 recipe
Calories: 256
Sodium: 303 mg
Cholesterol: 72 mg

Carbohydrate: trace
Protein: 35 gm
Fat: 12 gm

Heavenly Crab Cakes

Laura Letobar, Livonia, Michigan

When I switched to a low-fat diet, I thought I'd never be able to eat a crab cake again. But then I found this recipe. Now I can enjoy these little patties of paradise...without any guilt!

1 pound imitation crabmeat, flaked
1 cup Italian bread crumbs, *divided*
1/4 cup egg substitute
2 tablespoons fat-free mayonnaise
2 tablespoons Dijon mustard
1 tablespoon dill weed
1 tablespoon lime juice
1 teaspoon lemon juice
1 teaspoon Worcestershire sauce

Combine crabmeat, 1/2 cup of the bread crumbs, egg substitute, mayonnaise, mustard, dill, lime and lemon juices and Worcestershire sauce. Shape into eight patties. Place remaining bread crumbs in a shallow bowl; dredge each patty in crumbs to cover. Refrigerate for 30 minutes. In a large skillet coated with nonstick cooking spray, cook patties over medium heat until browned on both sides. **Yield:** 8 servings.

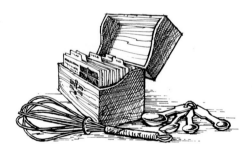

Exchanges: 1-1/2 Lean Meat, 1 Starch
Nutritional Information
Serving Size: 1 crab cake
Calories: 150
Sodium: 653 mg
Cholesterol: 14 mg

Carbohydrate: 22 gm
Protein: 11 gm
Fat: 2 gm

Lime Broiled Catfish

Nick Nicholson, Clarksdale, Mississippi

*To serve a reduced-calorie dish that is ready in about 15 minutes,
I came up with this fast recipe. I think the lime juice
adds a fresh flavor to the mild taste of the fish.*

**1 tablespoon margarine
2 tablespoons lime juice
1/4 teaspoon pepper
1/4 teaspoon garlic powder
2 catfish fillets (6 ounces *each*)**

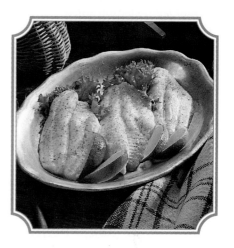

Melt margarine in a saucepan. Stir in lime juice, pepper and garlic powder; mix well. Remove from the heat and set aside. Place fillets in a shallow baking dish. Brush each generously with lime sauce. Broil for 5-8 minutes or until fish flakes easily with a fork. Remove to a warm serving dish; spoon pan juices over each fillet. **Yield:** 2 servings.

Exchanges: 4 Lean Meat, 1 Fat
Nutritional Information

Serving Size: 1 fillet
Calories: 254
Sodium: 156 mg
Cholesterol: 98 mg

Carbohydrate: 2 gm
Protein: 31 gm
Fat: 14 gm

Steamed Fish and Vegetables

Marilyn Newcomer, Menifee, California

*Everyone who tries this dish is amazed at how simple it is to prepare.
Plus it's tasty and low in fat. Best of all, this recipe can be easily doubled.*

1 whitefish fillet (4 ounces)
1/2 cup thinly sliced carrot
1/2 cup thinly sliced zucchini
2 teaspoons lemon juice
1/2 teaspoon dried parsley flakes
1/2 teaspoon lemon-pepper seasoning
1/4 teaspoon dill weed

Place fish on a 15-in. x 12-in. piece of heavy-duty foil. Add the vegetables and sprinkle with lemon juice, parsley, lemon pepper and dill. Fold foil over and fold in edges twice, forming a pouch. Place on a baking sheet. Bake at 450° for 15-20 minutes or until vegetables are tender and fish flakes easily with a fork. Carefully open pouch to allow steam to escape. **Yield:** 1 serving.

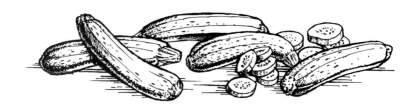

Exchanges: 3 Lean Meat, 1 Vegetable
Nutritional Information

Serving Size: 1 recipe
Calories: 226
Sodium: 768 mg
Cholesterol: 78 mg

Carbohydrate: 11 gm
Protein: 23 gm
Fat: 10 gm

Creole Jambalaya

Ruby Williams, Bogalusa, Louisiana

Jambalaya is a traditional Louisiana dish, coming from our Spanish and French culture. Rice is the main ingredient, with different meats or seafood mixed in. I particularly like this variation with shrimp and ham.

3/4 cup chopped onion
1/2 cup chopped celery
1/4 cup chopped green pepper
  2 garlic cloves, minced
  2 tablespoons margarine
  2 cups cubed fully cooked ham
  1 can (28 ounces) low-sodium
    tomatoes with liquid, cut up
2/3 cup low-sodium beef broth
  1 cup uncooked long grain white
    rice
  1 cup water
  1 teaspoon sugar
  1 teaspoon dried thyme
1/2 teaspoon chili powder
1/4 teaspoon pepper
1-1/2 pounds fresh *or* frozen
    uncooked shrimp, peeled and
    deveined
  1 tablespoon chopped fresh parsley

In a Dutch oven, saute onion, celery, green pepper and garlic in margarine until tender. Add next nine ingredients; bring to a boil. Reduce heat; cover and simmer until rice is tender, about 25 minutes. Add shrimp and parsley; simmer, uncovered, until shrimp are cooked, 7-10 minutes. **Yield:** 8 servings.

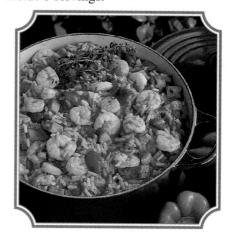

Exchanges: 3 Lean Meat, 1-1/2 Starch, 1 Vegetable
Nutritional Information
Serving Size: 1/8 recipe
Calories: 310
Sodium: 464 mg
Cholesterol: 154 mg

Carbohydrate: 28 gm
Protein: 31 gm
Fat: 8 gm

Greek Grilled Catfish

Rita Futral, Ocean Springs, Mississippi

Temperatures here on the Gulf Coast are moderate year-round, so we grill out a lot. My husband, Larry, came up with this recipe by experimenting. Our whole family likes the unique taste of this dish.

6 catfish fillets (8 ounces *each*)
Greek seasoning to taste
4 ounces feta cheese, crumbled
1 tablespoon dried mint
2 tablespoons olive oil

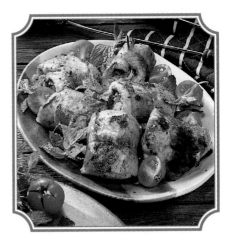

Sprinkle both sides of fillets with Greek seasoning. Sprinkle each fillet with 1 rounded tablespoon feta cheese and 1/2 teaspoon mint. Drizzle 1 teaspoon olive oil over each. Roll up fillets and secure with toothpicks. Grill over medium coals for 20-25 minutes or until fish flakes easily with a fork. Or, place fillets in a greased baking dish and bake at 350° for 30-35 minutes or until fish flakes easily with a fork. **Yield:** 6 servings.

Exchanges: 4-1/2 Lean Meat, 1 Fat

Nutritional Information

Serving Size: 1 fillet
Calories: 288
Sodium: 319 mg
Cholesterol: 115 mg

Carbohydrate: 1 gm
Protein: 34 gm
Fat: 16 gm

Meatless Meals

These pasta, pizza, egg and breakfast recipes deliciously prove that meatless meals don't have to be mediocre.

Mock Pasta Alfredo

Ruby Williams, Bogalusa, Louisiana

This recipe cuts the fat in alfredo sauce without sacrificing flavor. So if you've been yearning for pasta in a creamy sauce, indulge yourself with this dish.

1-1/2 cups low-fat cottage cheese
1/2 cup skim milk
2 garlic cloves, minced
2 tablespoons all-purpose flour
1 tablespoon lemon juice
1 teaspoon dried basil
1/2 teaspoon dry mustard
1/2 teaspoon pepper
8 ounces corkscrew noodles, cooked and drained
1 to 2 tomatoes, seeded and chopped

In a blender or food processor, process cottage cheese, milk and garlic until smooth. Add flour, lemon juice, basil, mustard and pepper; process until well blended. Pour into a saucepan. Cook over medium heat until thickened. Do not boil. Serve over noodles; sprinkle with tomatoes. **Yield:** 4 servings.

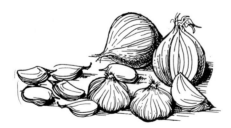

Exchanges: 2-1/2 Starch, 2 Lean Meat, 1 Vegetable

Nutritional Information

Serving Size: 1/4 recipe
Calories: 316
Sodium: 368 mg
Cholesterol: 8 mg

Carbohydrate: 53 gm
Protein: 20 gm
Fat: 2 gm

Tomato Pizza

Lois McAtee, Oceanside, California

My children liked to eat pizza with a lot of toppings, so I developed this recipe. We still make it often, even though the kids are grown. It's a delightful change from usual meat-topped pizza.

6 medium firm tomatoes, thinly sliced
1 large baked pizza crust (13 to 16 inches)
2 tablespoons olive oil
1 teaspoon salt
1 teaspoon pepper
1/2 cup diced green pepper
1/2 cup diced onion
1 tablespoon chopped fresh basil
1 cup (4 ounces) shredded low-fat mozzarella cheese
1 cup (4 ounces) shredded low-fat cheddar cheese

Place tomato slices in a circle on crust, overlapping slightly until crust is completely covered. Drizzle with olive oil. Season with salt and pepper. Cover with green pepper and onion. Sprinkle basil over all. Cover with mozzarella and cheddar cheeses. Bake at 400° for 15 minutes or until cheese is melted. Serve immediately. **Yield:** 8 servings.

REFRIGERATION RULE. It's best to store tomatoes at room temperature...refrigeration can ruin the flavor.

Exchanges: 1 Starch, 1 Meat, 1 Vegetable, 1 Fat

Nutritional Information

Serving Size: 1/8 recipe
Calories: 223
Sodium: 599 mg
Cholesterol: 22 mg

Carbohydrate: 21 gm
Protein: 12 gm
Fat: 12 gm

Cinnamon-Raisin Oatmeal

Rita Winterberger, Huson, Montana

This single-serving recipe is my favorite breakfast on cool mornings. It's hearty and very simple to prepare.

1/4 cup quick-cooking oats
1/4 cup Grape-Nuts cereal
1/4 cup raisins
1 teaspoon brown sugar
1 teaspoon ground cinnamon
1 cup skim milk

In a microwave-safe cereal bowl, combine all ingredients. Microwave on high for 3 minutes. **Yield:** 1 serving.

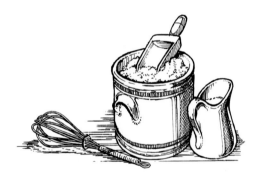

Exchanges: 3 Starch, 2 Fruit, 1 Skim Milk
Nutritional Information

Serving Size: 1 recipe
Calories: 395
Sodium: 325 mg
Cholesterol: 4 mg

Carbohydrate: 83 gm
Protein: 15 gm
Fat: 3 gm

Puffy Apple Omelet

Melissa Davenport, Campbell, Minnesota

I could make this omelet every day! I guess I consider it to be mostly a festive dish, but you could fix it anytime...including for a light supper.

3 tablespoons all-purpose flour
1/4 teaspoon baking powder
2 eggs, *separated*
3 tablespoons skim milk
3 tablespoons sugar
1 tablespoon lemon juice
TOPPING:
1 large baking apple, thinly
** sliced**
1 teaspoon sugar
1/4 teaspoon ground cinnamon

In a small bowl, combine flour and baking powder. Add egg yolks and milk; mix well and set aside. In a small mixing bowl, beat egg whites until foamy. Gradually add sugar, beating until stiff peaks form. Fold in yolk mixture and lemon juice. Pour into a greased 1-1/2-qt. shallow baking dish. Arrange apple slices on top. Combine sugar and cinnamon; sprinkle over all. Bake, uncovered, at 375° for 18-20 minutes or until a knife inserted near the center comes out clean. Serve immediately. **Yield:** 2 servings.

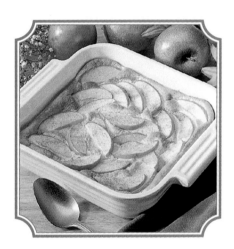

Exchanges: 1 Starch, 1 Meat, 1/2 Fruit

Nutritional Information

Serving Size: 1/2 recipe
Calories: 193
Sodium: 148 mg
Cholesterol: 214 mg

Carbohydrate: 26 gm
Protein: 9 gm
Fat: 6 gm

Applesauce Oatmeal Pancakes

Martha Cage, Wheeling, West Virginia

*My family just loves pancakes for breakfast. When I made this
slightly sweet variety, everyone kept asking for more!*

1 cup quick-cooking oats
1/4 cup whole wheat flour
1/4 cup all-purpose flour
1 tablespoon baking powder
1 cup skim milk
2 tablespoons Sugarless
   Applesauce (recipe on page 247)
   or purchased sugarless
   applesauce
4 egg whites

In a bowl, combine the oats, flours and
baking powder. In another bowl, combine milk, applesauce and egg whites;
add to dry ingredients and mix well. Pour
batter by 1/4 cupfuls onto a heated griddle coated with nonstick cooking spray.
Cook until bubbles appear on the top;
turn and cook until lightly browned.
Yield: 10 pancakes.

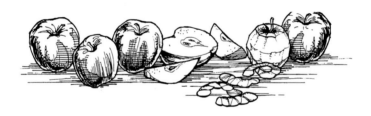

Exchanges: 1 Starch
Nutritional Information

Serving Size: 2 pancakes
Calories: 91
Sodium: 323 mg
Cholesterol: 1 mg

Carbohydrate: 15 gm
Protein: 5 gm
Fat: trace

Meatless Spaghetti

Barbara Njaa, Nikishka, Alaska

*This sauce is so chunky and good you'll think it has meat!
Folks will love this delicious main dish.*

6 garlic cloves, minced
1 cup chopped celery
1 medium *or* large onion, chopped
2 tablespoons cooking oil
6 small zucchini, chopped (about
  2 pounds)
1 green pepper, chopped
1 can (6 ounces) pitted ripe olives,
  drained and sliced
4 low-sodium beef bouillon cubes
1 cup hot water
1 jar (6 ounces) sliced
  mushrooms, drained
1 can (28 ounces) diced tomatoes
  with liquid
2 cans (15 ounces *each*) tomato
  sauce
1 can (6 ounces) tomato paste
2 teaspoons dried basil
2 teaspoons dried oregano
2 teaspoons dried parsley flakes
1/2 teaspoon pepper
Hot cooked noodles, optional

In a large saucepan or a Dutch oven, saute garlic, celery and onion in oil until tender. Add zucchini, green pepper and olives; saute for 2-3 minutes. Dissolve bouillon in water; add to vegetables. Add the next eight ingredients and bring to a boil. Reduce heat; cover and simmer for 1 hour, stirring occasionally. Serve over noodles if desired. **Yield:** 14 servings.

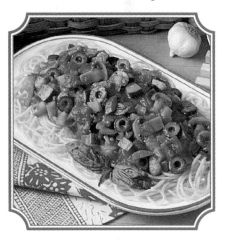

Exchanges: 3 Vegetable, 1 Fat

Nutritional Information

Serving Size: 1 cup sauce
Calories: 102
Sodium: 624 mg
Cholesterol: 0

Carbohydrate: 14 gm
Protein: 4 gm
Fat: 5 gm
(Calculated without noodles)

Country Breakfast Cereal

Sharon Skildum, Maple Grove, Minnesota

Store-bought cereals are packed with preservatives. But this hot, hearty homemade cereal is loaded with natural ingredients and fabulous flavor.

3 cups cooked brown rice
2 cups skim milk
1/2 cup raisins
1 tablespoon margarine
1 teaspoon ground cinnamon
1/8 teaspoon salt

In a large saucepan, combine rice, milk, raisins, margarine, cinnamon and salt. Bring to a boil, stirring occasionally. Reduce heat; cover and simmer for 8-10 minutes or until thickened. **Yield:** 6 servings.

> **RICE TO KNOW!** When refrigerating cooked rice, cover the container tightly so the grains don't dry out or absorb flavors of other foods.

Exchanges: 1 Starch, 1 Fruit, 1/2 Skim Milk, 1/2 Fat
Nutritional Information

Serving Size: 1/6 recipe
Calories: 197
Sodium: 110 mg
Cholesterol: 1 mg

Carbohydrate: 39 gm
Protein: 6 gm
Fat: 3 gm

Vegetable Quiche

Elnora Johnson, Union City, Tennessee

I've made and served this tasty dish for a long time.
It has a unique rice crust and really holds up well for cutting.

1-1/2 cups cooked brown rice, room
    temperature
  3/4 cup egg substitute, *divided*
  3/4 cup shredded low-fat
    mozzarella cheese, *divided*
1-1/2 cups chopped fresh broccoli
  3/4 cup sliced fresh mushrooms
  1/4 cup skim milk
    1 tablespoon margarine, melted

In a bowl, combine rice, 1/4 cup egg substitute and half of the cheese; mix well. Pat into the bottom and up the sides of a 9-in. pie plate coated with nonstick cooking spray; set aside. In another bowl, combine the broccoli, mushrooms, milk, margarine and remaining egg substitute. Pour into crust. Bake, uncovered, at 375° for 20-25 minutes or until a knife inserted near the center comes out clean. Sprinkle with the remaining cheese. Return to the oven until cheese melts. **Yield:** 8 servings.

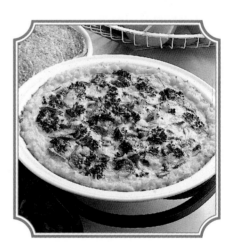

Exchanges: 1 Meat, 1 Vegetable, 1/2 Starch
Nutritional Information
Serving Size: 1/8 recipe   Carbohydrate: 13 gm
Calories: 131   Protein: 7 gm
Sodium: 119 mg   Fat: 6 gm
Cholesterol: 7 mg

Oat Pancakes

Linda Hicks, Pinconning, Michigan

My daughter brought this recipe home from school one day, and we loved it. Since then, these pancakes have been a regular part of Sunday morning breakfasts.

1 cup quick-cooking oats
1 cup all-purpose flour
2 tablespoons sugar
2 teaspoons baking powder
1 teaspoon salt
2 eggs, lightly beaten
1-1/2 cups skim milk
1/4 cup vegetable oil
1 teaspoon lemon juice
Low-sugar maple syrup, optional

Combine oats, flour, sugar, baking powder and salt in a mixing bowl. Make a well in the center. Combine eggs, milk, oil and lemon juice; pour into well and stir just until moistened. Pour batter by 1/4 cupfuls onto a lightly greased hot griddle; turn when bubbles form on top of pancakes. Cook until second side is golden brown. Serve with syrup if desired. **Yield:** 12 pancakes.

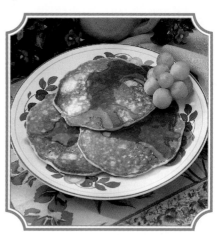

Exchanges: 1–1/2 Starch, 1 Fat, 1/2 Skim Milk

Nutritional Information

Serving Size: 2 pancakes
Calories: 241
Sodium: 581 mg
Cholesterol: 71 mg

Carbohydrate: 25 gm
Protein: 8 gm
Fat: 12 gm
(Calculated without syrup)

Baked Macaroni and Cheese

Lois McAtee, Oceanside, California

This recipe proves you can watch your diet and still enjoy down–home country cooking. The blend of seasonings and cheeses give this hearty casserole great flavor.

1 tablespoon margarine
3 tablespoons all-purpose flour
2 cups skim milk
3/4 to 1 teaspoon dried marjoram
1/2 teaspoon dried thyme
1/8 teaspoon ground nutmeg
1/8 teaspoon paprika
1 tablespoon Dijon mustard
1/2 cup grated Parmesan cheese, *divided*
1 box (7 ounces) elbow macaroni, cooked and drained
1 cup low-fat cottage cheese

Melt margarine in a large saucepan. Add flour and stir to form a smooth paste. Gradually add milk, stirring constantly. Bring to a boil; boil 1 minute or until thickened. Add marjoram, thyme, nutmeg and paprika; stir to blend. Remove from the heat. Stir in mustard and 1/3 cup Parmesan cheese; mix well. Add macaroni and cottage cheese; toss to coat. Pour into an 8-in. square baking dish sprayed with nonstick cooking spray. Sprinkle with remaining Parmesan. Bake, uncovered, at 350° for 30 minutes or until heated through and top is golden brown. **Yield:** 4 servings.

Exchanges: 3 Starch, 2 Meat

Nutritional Information

Serving Size: 1/4 recipe
Calories: 367
Sodium: 530 mg
Cholesterol: 13 mg

Carbohydrate: 50 gm
Protein: 23 gm
Fat: 8 gm

Homemade Egg Substitute

Anita Freed, Portage, Michigan

I really enjoy egg dishes, but I have to watch how many I eat. This recipe is easy to whip up anytime plus it tastes better than prepackaged egg substitute products. I use this whenever a recipe calls for egg substitute.

2 egg whites
2 teaspoons nonfat dry milk solids
1 teaspoon canola *or* corn oil
1 drop yellow food coloring

In a small bowl, combine all ingredients; mix well. Use as a substitute for 1 egg. **Yield:** 1 serving.

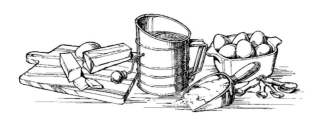

Exchanges: 1-1/2 Meat

Nutritional Information

Serving Size: 1 recipe
Calories: 90
Sodium: 127 mg
Cholesterol: 1 mg

Carbohydrate: 3 gm
Protein: 9 gm
Fat: 5 gm

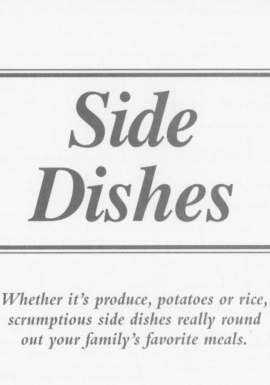

Side Dishes

Whether it's produce, potatoes or rice, scrumptious side dishes really round out your family's favorite meals.

Green Bean Medley

Janice Cox, Smithfield, Kentucky

*With its fresh taste and hint of savory, this quick and easy
side dish is sure to complement all of your main meals.
I always seem to have the ingredients for this recipe on hand.*

1-1/2 pounds fresh green beans,
  halved
  1 medium onion, thinly sliced into
    rings
  1 celery rib, sliced
  2 to 3 carrots, cut into 2-inch
    strips
  2 to 3 tablespoons minced fresh
    savory *or* 2 to 3 teaspoons dried
    savory
  1/8 teaspoon pepper
  1 cup water

In a large saucepan, combine all ingredients; bring to a boil. Reduce heat; cover and simmer for 5-10 minutes or until vegetables are tender, stirring occasionally. Remove with a slotted spoon to a serving bowl. **Yield:** 6 servings.

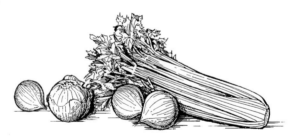

Exchanges: 1-1/2 Vegetable
Nutritional Information

Serving Size: 1 cup
Calories: 41
Sodium: 20 mg
Cholesterol: 0

Carbohydrate: 9 gm
Protein: 2 gm
Fat: trace

Squash and Broccoli Stir-Fry

Erlene Cornelius, Spring City, Tennessee

The first summer that my husband and I were retired, we had an abundance of squash. I was raised on a farm and taught nothing should go to waste, so I hunted in my recipe file and found this one. I've made it often ever since.

1 tablespoon lemon juice
2 teaspoons honey
2 tablespoons cooking oil
1 pound butternut squash, peeled, seeded and cut into 1/4-inch slices
1 garlic clove, minced
1/4 teaspoon ground ginger
1 cup fresh broccoli florets
1/2 cup bias-sliced celery
1/2 cup thinly sliced onion
2 tablespoons sunflower seeds

Combine lemon juice and honey; set aside. In a wok or large skillet, heat oil on medium-high. Add squash, garlic and ginger. Stir-fry about 3 minutes. Add the broccoli, celery and onion; stir-fry 3-4 minutes or until crisp-tender. Remove from heat and quickly toss with the honey mixture. Sprinkle with sunflower seeds. Serve immediately. **Yield:** 6 servings.

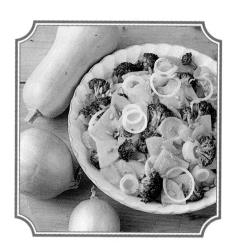

Exchanges: 2 Vegetable, 1-1/2 Fat

Nutritional Information

Serving Size: 1/6 recipe
Calories: 113
Sodium: 20 mg
Cholesterol: 0

Carbohydrate: 13 gm
Protein: 2 gm
Fat: 7 gm

Scalloped Potatoes for One

Alvena Franklin, Coldwater, Michigan

As a widow, I cook for myself much of the time and have learned to scale down recipes that I often served when our four kids were still at home. This recipe makes just the right amount.

1 small potato, peeled and
  sliced (about 1/2 cup)
1/3 cup skim milk
1 small garlic clove, minced
1/8 teaspoon pepper
1/2 teaspoon margarine, melted
1 to 2 tablespoons shredded
  cheddar cheese

In a small saucepan, combine potato slices, milk, garlic and pepper; bring to a boil. Coat 10-oz. custard cup with melted margarine. Pour potato mixture into dish. Sprinkle with cheese. Bake, uncovered, at 375° for 35 minutes or until potatoes are tender. **Yield:** 1 serving.

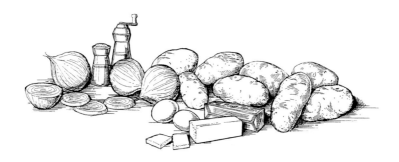

Exchanges: 1 Starch, 1/2 Meat, 1/2 Fat, 1/2 Skim Milk

Nutritional Information

Serving Size: 1 recipe
Calories: 179
Sodium: 131 mg
Cholesterol: 12 mg

Carbohydrate: 24 gm
Protein: 8 gm
Fat: 6 gm

Zesty Zucchini Skillet

Barbara Winders, Spencer, Indiana

In our family, we all like zucchini, so I'm always trying to find some new ways to prepare it. This has been one of my most-requested recipes for a number of years.

2 tablespoons cooking oil
4 cups diced zucchini
1 cup chopped onion
1 cup chopped carrots
1/2 green pepper, thinly sliced
3/4 cup chopped celery
1/2 teaspoon garlic powder
2 teaspoons dried basil
2 teaspoons dried oregano
1/4 teaspoon salt
Pepper to taste
1/3 cup picante sauce
2 teaspoons prepared mustard
1 medium tomato, diced
1/2 cup shredded Monterey Jack cheese

In a skillet, heat oil over medium. Cook and stir the next six ingredients until vegetables are crisp-tender. Combine basil, oregano, salt, pepper, picante sauce and mustard; pour into skillet. Cook and stir for 3 minutes. Gently stir in tomatoes; heat through. Sprinkle with cheese and serve immediately. **Yield:** 8 servings.

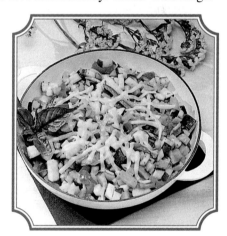

Exchanges: 1-1/2 Vegetable, 1 Fat

Nutritional Information

Serving Size: 1/8 recipe
Calories: 83
Sodium: 162 mg
Cholesterol: 8 mg

Carbohydrate: 6 gm
Protein: 3 gm
Fat: 6 gm

Savory Peas

Claire Talone, Morrisville, Pennsylvania

I came up with this recipe one day when I wanted to add some "zip" to plain peas. This recipe did the trick! Everyone commented on the great flavor and festive color.

2 tablespoons margarine
1 package (10 ounces) frozen
  peas, thawed
1 cup sliced celery
1/2 cup chopped onion
1 tablespoon minced fresh
  savory *or* 1-1/2 teaspoons
  dried savory
2 tablespoons diced pimientos

Melt margarine in a heavy saucepan; add the next four ingredients. Cover and cook over medium heat for 6-8 minutes or until vegetables are tender. Stir in pimientos. **Yield:** 6 servings.

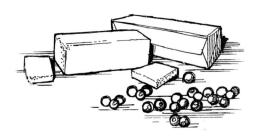

Exchanges: 1 Fat, 1/2 Starch
Nutritional Information

Serving Size: 1/2 cup
Calories: 74
Sodium: 93 mg
Cholesterol: 0

Carbohydrate: 8 gm
Protein: 2 gm
Fat: 4 gm

German Red Cabbage

Jeannette Heim, Concord, California

Sunday afternoons were a time for family gatherings when I was a child. While the uncles played cards, the aunts prepared wonderful German treats such as this traditional red cabbage.

1 medium onion, sliced
1 unpeeled apple, cored and
  sliced
1 medium head red cabbage,
  shredded
Artificial sweetener equivalent to 1/3
  cup sugar
1/3 cup white *or* cider vinegar
1/4 teaspoon pepper

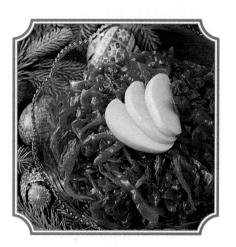

In a large Dutch oven coated with non-stick cooking spray, saute onion and apple until tender. Add all remaining ingredients. Cover and cook until tender, about 1 hour. Serve hot or cold. **Yield:** 10 servings.

Exchanges: 1-1/2 Vegetable

Nutritional Information

Serving Size: 1/10 recipe
Calories: 43
Sodium: 1 mg
Cholesterol: 0

Carbohydrate: 10 gm
Protein: 2 gm
Fat: less than 1 gm

Corn Medley

Ruth Andrewson, Leavenworth, Washington

This garden-fresh medley showcases corn in a colorful blend with tomato, green pepper and onion, while cumin adds a little spark. It's one of my favorite recipes when corn's in season.

**2 cups fresh-cut sweet corn
  (3 to 4 ears)
2 tablespoons light margarine
1/4 cup chopped onion
1/4 cup chopped green pepper
1/4 teaspoon ground cumin
1 large tomato, chopped and
  seeded
Artificial sweetener equivalent to 2
  tablespoons sugar**

Combine the first five ingredients in a medium saucepan; cook and stir over medium heat until margarine is melted. Cover and cook over low heat for 10 minutes. Stir in tomato and sweetener; cook, covered, 5 minutes longer. **Yield:** 5 servings.

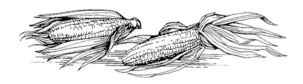

Exchanges: 1 Starch, 1 Fat
Nutritional Information

Serving Size: 2/3 cup
Calories: 96
Sodium: 71 mg
Cholesterol: 0

Carbohydrate: 14 gm
Protein: 2 gm
Fat: 4 gm

Gingered Carrots

Mary Dennis, Bryan, Ohio

I first made this original recipe some 40 years ago, and it hasn't failed me yet. The thing I like about it is that it isn't plain. The flavorings dress up an "ordinary vegetable".

5 to 6 carrots, peeled and cut into chunks
1/2 teaspoon ground ginger
1 teaspoon sugar
1/4 cup margarine
2 tablespoons chopped fresh parsley

In a skillet, cook carrots in a small amount of water until almost tender. Drain. Add ginger, sugar and margarine; heat over low until carrots are warm and coated with the sauce. Sprinkle with parsley. Serve immediately. **Yield:** 4 servings.

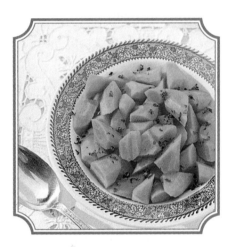

Exchanges: 1-1/2 Vegetable, 1-1/2 Fat

Nutritional Information

Serving Size: 1/4 recipe
Calories: 107
Sodium: 94 mg
Cholesterol: 0

Carbohydrate: 13 gm
Protein: 2 gm
Fat: 7 gm

Italian Zucchini

Christopher Gordon, Springfield, Missouri

When I met my wife, I found she didn't particularly like to spend time in the kitchen. Now I enjoy planning menus and cooking for the both of us. This nice hot vegetable dish is one I frequently prepare.

4 cups sliced zucchini
1 medium onion, sliced into rings
2 medium tomatoes, sliced
1 lemon, quartered
1-1/2 teaspoons Italian seasoning
3/4 teaspoon crushed red pepper flakes
1 tablespoon margarine

In a 2-1/2-qt. casserole coated with non-stick cooking spray, layer one-third of the zucchini, onion and tomatoes. Squeeze one lemon quarter over all. Sprinkle with 1/2 teaspoon Italian seasoning and 1/4 teaspoon red pepper flakes. Repeat layers. Dot with margarine. Squeeze remaining lemon over all. Cover and bake at 350° for 1 hour or until vegetables are tender. Serve immediately. **Yield:** 4 servings.

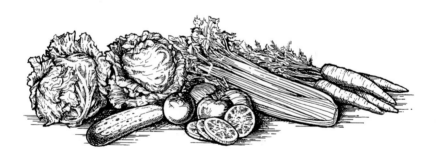

Exchanges: 1-1/2 Vegetable, 1/2 Fat
Nutritional Information

Serving Size: 1/4 recipe
Calories: 64
Sodium: 35 mg
Cholesterol: 0

Carbohydrate: 9 gm
Protein: 2 gm
Fat: 3 gm

Southern Okra

Bobbie Jo Yokley, Franklin, Kentucky

This recipe dates back generations in my family. I enjoy it so much because I can use the fresh vegetables that are so abundant here in the South. But I know you'll love this dish no matter where you live!

1 tablespoon sugar
1 teaspoon all-purpose flour
1/2 teaspoon salt
1/2 teaspoon pepper
2 cups sliced fresh okra
Boiling water
2 tablespoons vegetable oil
1 medium onion, chopped
1 medium green pepper, chopped
3 medium tomatoes, peeled and chopped
Hot cooked rice, optional

Combine the first four ingredients; set aside. In a covered saucepan, cook okra in boiling water for 10 minutes or until tender. Drain and set aside. In a skillet, heat oil over medium. Saute onion and green pepper until tender. Stir in sugar mixture and tomatoes; cook for 5 minutes. Add okra and simmer until heated through, stirring as little as possible. Serve with rice if desired. **Yield:** 6 servings.

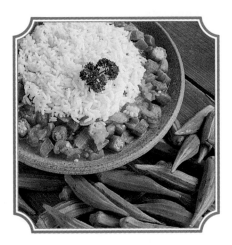

Exchanges: 1-1/2 Vegetable, 1 Fat

Nutritional Information

Serving Size: 1/6 recipe
Calories: 83
Sodium: 333 mg
Cholesterol: 0

Carbohydrate: 11 gm
Protein: 2 gm
Fat: 5 gm
(Calculated without rice)

Broccoli with Red Pepper

Karen Davies, Wanipigow, Manitoba

*This simple-to-prepare side dish gets its great flavor
from the crunchy water chestnuts. I think you'll
especially like the touch of color it brings to your table.*

2 tablespoons vegetable oil
4 cups broccoli florets
2 teaspoons minced fresh
   gingerroot
2 garlic cloves, minced
1 sweet red pepper, cut into strips
1 can (8 ounces) sliced
   water chestnuts, drained

In a skillet, heat oil over high. Stir-fry broccoli, ginger and garlic until broccoli is crisp-tender, about 2 minutes. Add red pepper and water chestnuts; stir-fry just until heated through, about 1 minute. Serve immediately. **Yield:** 4 servings.

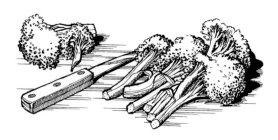

Exchanges: 2 Vegetable, 1-1/2 Fat
Nutritional Information

Serving Size: 1/4 recipe
Calories: 117
Sodium: 28 mg
Cholesterol: 0

Carbohydrate: 17 gm
Protein: 3 gm
Fat: 7 gm

Potato Pancakes

Roseanna Budell, Dunnellon, Florida

We grew our own potatoes on the small farm in New Hampshire where I was raised. These pancakes are very good served with any pork dish. But I've also been known to serve them as a meal by themselves.

**3 cups finely shredded peeled
   potatoes, well drained
2 eggs, well beaten
1-1/2 tablespoons all-purpose flour
1/8 teaspoon baking powder
1/2 teaspoon grated onion**

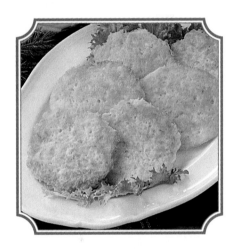

In a mixing bowl, gently combine potatoes and eggs. Combine flour, baking powder and onion; stir into potato mixture. Drop by tablespoonfuls onto a preheated nonstick skillet coated with nonstick cooking spray. Brown lightly on both sides. Serve with applesauce or syrup if desired. **Yield:** 12 (2-inch) pancakes.

Exchanges: 1 Starch

Nutritional Information

Serving Size: 1 pancake
Calories: 77
Sodium: 21 mg
Cholesterol: 36 mg

Carbohydrate: 15 gm
Protein: 3 gm
Fat: 1 gm

Mashed Potato for One

Winifred Chesborough, Truth or Consequences, New Mexico

With cream cheese and dill, these comforting mashed potatoes are so creamy and delicious. Plus, this recipe can be easily doubled when cooking for a larger group. I hope you enjoy it!

1 medium potato, peeled and
  cooked
2 tablespoons skim milk
1 tablespoon light cream
  cheese, softened
1 teaspoon margarine
1/8 teaspoon snipped fresh dill *or*
  pinch dill weed
Dash pepper

In a small bowl, mash all ingredients until smooth. Spoon into a small microwave-safe dish. Cook on high for 1 minute or until heated through. **Yield:** 1 serving.

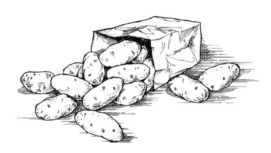

Exchanges: 1-1/2 Starch, 1 Fat
Nutritional Information

Serving Size: 1 recipe
Calories: 163
Sodium: 134 mg
Cholesterol: 9 mg

Carbohydrate: 22 gm
Protein: 5 gm
Fat: 6 gm

Marinated Grilled Vegetables

Marian Platt, Sequim, Washington

*We camp out often in summer and do a lot of cooking over charcoal…
meats and vegetables included! This recipe contains some of my
family's favorite veggies, so this dish always disappears quickly.*

6 small onions, halved
**4 carrots, cut into 1-1/2-inch
   chunks**
1/3 cup olive *or* vegetable oil
**1/2 teaspoon dried rosemary,
   crushed**
1/4 teaspoon dried marjoram
Dash pepper
**6 small pattypan *or* sunburst
   squash**
**1 medium zucchini, cut into
   1-inch chunks**
**1 medium green pepper, cut into
   1-inch pieces**
**1 medium sweet red pepper, cut
   into 1-inch pieces**

In a saucepan, cook onions and carrots in
water for 10 minutes or until crisp-tender;
drain. In a large bowl, combine oil and
seasonings; add all of the vegetables and
mix well. Cover and refrigerate for at least
1 hour. Drain, reserving marinade. Thread
vegetables alternately onto skewers. Grill,
uncovered, over medium coals for 15-20
minutes or until tender. Turn and baste
with the marinade every 5 minutes. **Yield:**
6 servings.

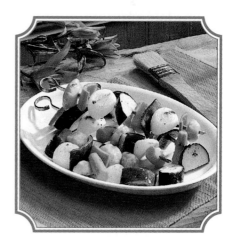

Exchanges: 2 Vegetable, 1 Fat

Nutritional Information

Serving Size: 1/6 recipe
Calories: 97
Sodium: 28 mg
Cholesterol: 0

Carbohydrate: 11 gm
Protein: 2 gm
Fat: 6 gm

Fresh Vegetable Stew

Carol Fischer, Pewaukee, Wisconsin

Sunny, colorful and brimming with garden flavor, this easy stovetop dish stirs in several different squashes along with other favorite veggies. Why not serve it with your best main meal tonight?

1 large onion, sliced
3 garlic cloves, minced
1 tablespoon olive oil
1 pound yellow squash, cut into 1/2-inch cubes
1 pound pattypan squash, cut into 1/2-inch cubes
2 medium tomatoes, peeled and chopped
3/4 pound fresh green beans, cut into 1-inch pieces

1-1/4 cups fresh sweet corn
1/4 teaspoon pepper

In a large skillet, saute onion and garlic in oil until tender. Add squash, tomatoes and beans. Reduce heat; cover and simmer 15 minutes or until squash is tender. Add corn and pepper. Cook for 3 minutes or until corn is tender. **Yield:** 12 servings.

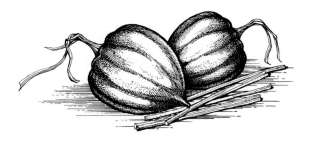

Exchanges: 2 Vegetable

Nutritional Information

Serving Size: 2/3 cup
Calories: 59
Sodium: 184 mg
Cholesterol: 0

Carbohydrate: 11 gm
Protein: 2 gm
Fat: 2 gm

Continental Zucchini

Martha Fehl, Brookville, Indiana

Zucchini are big and plentiful here, and people often joke about using them up before they multiply! This colorful, easy recipe wins raves at church gatherings.

1 tablespoon cooking oil
1 pound zucchini (about 3 small), cubed
1 to 2 garlic cloves, minced
1 jar (2 ounces) chopped pimientos, drained
1 can (15-1/2 ounces) whole kernel corn, drained
1/4 teaspoon lemon-pepper seasoning
1/2 cup shredded low-fat mozzarella cheese

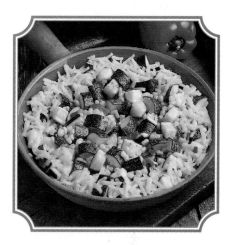

Heat oil in a large skillet. Saute zucchini and garlic for 3-4 minutes. Add pimientos, corn and lemon pepper; cook and stir for 2-3 minutes or until zucchini is tender. Sprinkle with cheese and heat until cheese melts. **Yield:** 6 servings.

Exchanges: 1 Vegetable, 1 Meat, 1/2 Starch
Nutritional Information

Serving Size: 1/6 recipe
Calories: 131
Sodium: 107 mg
Cholesterol: 10 mg

Carbohydrate: 15 gm
Protein: 8 gm
Fat: 6 gm

Ground Beef Dressing

Lynn Ireland, Lebanon, Wisconsin

As is true with most families, food is an important part of all our celebrations. But I like to make special-occasion meals as nutritious—and tasty—as possible. That's why I know everyone at your table will savor this delicious dressing.

1 pound extra-lean ground beef
1 medium onion, chopped
1 medium apple, chopped
2 celery ribs, chopped
8 cups bread cubes
1 tablespoon poultry seasoning
1/2 teaspoon pepper
2 cups low-sodium chicken
   broth

In a skillet, brown beef; drain. Place in a large bowl; add remaining ingredients and mix well. Transfer to a 3-qt. baking dish that has been coated with nonstick cooking spray. Cover and bake at 325° for 1-1/2 hours. Uncover and bake 10 minutes more or until the dressing is lightly browned. **Yield:** 16 servings.

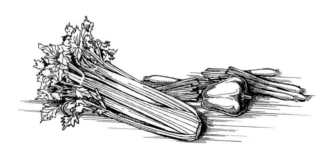

Exchanges: 2 Starch, 2 Lean Meat

Nutritional Information

Serving Size: 3/4 cup
Calories: 272
Sodium: 414 mg
Cholesterol: 18 mg

Carbohydrate: 39 gm
Protein: 14 gm
Fat: 6 gm

Herbed Rice Pilaf

Norma Poole, Auburndale, Florida

*The zesty flavor of onion is great with the crunch of celery in this recipe.
It's a tasty side dish for any meal. I sometimes add chopped
shrimp, chicken or beef to make it into a one-dish meal.*

2 cups uncooked long grain rice
1 cup chopped celery
1/2 cup chopped onion
1/4 cup margarine
4 cups low-sodium chicken broth
1 teaspoon Worcestershire sauce
1 teaspoon light soy sauce
1 teaspoon dried oregano
1 teaspoon dried thyme

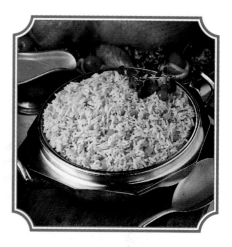

In a skillet, saute rice, celery and onion in margarine until the rice is lightly browned and the vegetables are tender. Spoon into a greased 2-qt. casserole. Combine all remaining ingredients; pour over rice mixture. Cover and bake at 325° for 50 minutes or until the rice is done. **Yield:** 8 servings.

Exchanges: 1 Starch, 1 Vegetable, 1/2 Fat

Nutritional Information

Serving Size: 1/8 recipe
Calories: 124
Sodium: 65 mg
Cholesterol: 0

Carbohydrate: 21 gm
Protein: 2 gm
Fat: 3 gm

French Peas

John Davis, Mobile, Alabama

It's always nice to have a side dish recipe that complements any meal—and that's no fuss to prepare. This tasty medley of peas, mushrooms and onion is sure to satisfy.

1 teaspoon margarine
2 teaspoons water
2 medium fresh mushrooms,
  thinly sliced
1/2 cup frozen peas
2 thin onion slices

Melt margarine in a small saucepan; add all remaining ingredients. Cover and cook until the peas are tender, stirring occasionally. **Yield:** 1 serving.

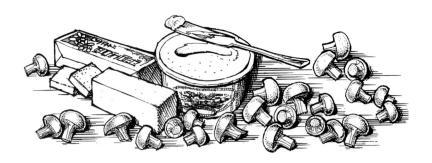

Exchanges: 1 Starch, 1 Fat
Nutritional Information

Serving Size: 1 recipe
Calories: 104
Sodium: 104 mg
Cholesterol: 0

Carbohydrate: 13 gm
Protein: 4 gm
Fat: 1 gm

Pumpkin Vegetable Stew

Gerald Knudsen, Quincy, Massachusetts

I created this stew as a way to use pumpkins for more than just breads and pies. It's a hearty side dish for meat and potatoes. It's great during the fall, and is as colorful as the season. My family loves it.

4 cups cubed peeled pumpkin
   or winter squash
1 can (14-1/2 ounces) tomatoes
   with liquid, cut up
1/2 cup low-sodium chicken broth
2 cups fresh cut green beans
   (1-inch pieces)
1 cup fresh *or* frozen corn
1/2 cup sliced onion
1/2 cup chopped green pepper
1 garlic clove, minced
1/2 teaspoon chili powder
1/4 teaspoon pepper

In a large saucepan, combine all the ingredients. Bring to a boil. Reduce heat; cover and simmer for 40-45 minutes or until the vegetables are tender. **Yield:** 6 servings.

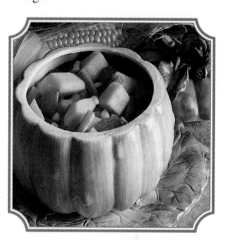

Exchanges: 1 Starch, 1 Vegetable
Nutritional Information

Serving Size: 1-1/3 cups
Calories: 83
Sodium: 109 mg
Cholesterol: trace

Carbohydrate: 20 gm
Protein: 4 gm
Fat: 1 gm

Garden Vegetable Medley

Suzanne Pelegrin, Ocala, Florida

This recipe combines a variety of fresh produce that's perfect on hot summer nights. My family looks forward to this dish often when the vegetables are in season.

1 medium yellow summer
   squash
1 medium zucchini
1 medium onion, halved
1 medium green pepper
3 garlic cloves, minced
1-1/2 teaspoons minced fresh
   oregano *or* 1/2 teaspoon
   dried oregano
1-1/2 teaspoons minced fresh basil
   or 1/2 teaspoon dried basil
1/2 cup low-sodium chicken broth
2 cups cherry tomatoes, halved

Cut vegetables into 2-in. x 1/2-in. strips. In a skillet or wok, simmer vegetables, garlic and seasonings in broth over medium heat. Stir constantly until crisp-tender, about 7 minutes. Add tomatoes and heat through. Serve immediately. **Yield:** 8 servings.

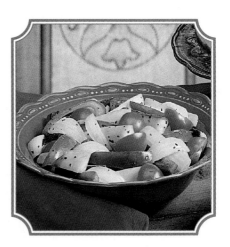

Exchanges: 1-1/2 Vegetable

Nutritional Information

Serving Size: 3/4 cup
Calories: 36
Sodium: 11 mg
Cholesterol: 0

Carbohydrate: 8 gm
Protein: 2 gm
Fat: trace

Sugarless Applesauce

Margery Bryan, Royal City, Washington

A friend gave me this delicious recipe 20 years ago, and I've made applesauce this way ever since. We grow a lot of apples in this area and have fun putting this crop to good use.

8 cups sliced peeled tart apples
1/2 to 1 can (12 ounces) diet white soda
1/2 to 1 teaspoon ground cinnamon

In a saucepan over medium heat, cook apples, soda and cinnamon until apples are tender, about 45 minutes. Serve warm or cold. **Yield:** 8 servings.

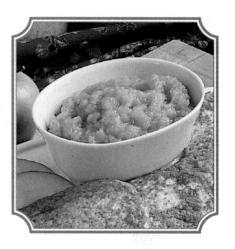

TASTY TIP. This makes a great side dish or topping for pancakes or waffles. You can also use this applesauce in the Applesauce Oatmeal Pancakes recipe on page 218.

Exchanges: 1 Fruit

Nutritional Information

Serving Size: 1/2 cup
Calories: 74
Sodium: 1 mg
Cholesterol: 0

Carbohydrate: 19 gm
Protein: trace
Fat: trace

Skillet Seasoned Rice

John Davis, Mobile, Alabama

*I recently put together a special cookbook for folks who cook for themselves.
One of my favorite recipes inside the book is this nicely seasoned rice.*

1/4 cup uncooked long grain rice
1 green onion with top, cut into
   1-inch pieces
1 tablespoon margarine
1/8 teaspoon *each* dried tarragon,
   thyme, basil, parsley flakes
   and pepper
1/2 cup low-sodium chicken broth

In a small saucepan, cook rice and onion in margarine until onion is tender. Add the seasonings; cook for 1 minute. Add broth; bring to a boil. Cover and simmer for 15 minutes or until liquid is absorbed and rice is tender. **Yield:** 1 serving.

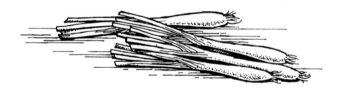

Exchanges: 2-1/2 Starch, 2 Fat

Nutritional Information

Serving Size: 1 recipe
Calories: 284
Sodium: 129 mg
Cholesterol: 0

Carbohydrate: 39 gm
Protein: 5 gm
Fat: 12 gm

Broccoli-Mushroom Medley

Cherie Sechrist, Red Lion, Pennsylvania

People will think you fussed over this fresh flavorful vegetable dish, but really it's quite simple. I make this often when time gets away from me and the family's ready for dinner.

1-1/2 pounds fresh broccoli, cut into florets
1 teaspoon lemon juice
1 teaspoon sugar
1 teaspoon cornstarch
1/4 teaspoon ground nutmeg
1 cup sliced fresh mushrooms
1 medium onion, sliced into rings
1 to 2 garlic cloves, minced
3 tablespoons cooking oil

Steam broccoli for 1-2 minutes or until crisp-tender. Rinse in cold water and set aside. In a bowl, combine lemon juice, sugar, cornstarch and nutmeg; set aside. In a large skillet or wok over high heat, stir-fry mushrooms, onion and garlic in oil for 3 minutes. Add broccoli and lemon juice mixture; stir-fry for 1-2 minutes. Serve immediately. **Yield:** 6 servings.

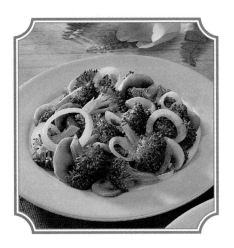

Exchanges: 2 Vegetable, 1 Fat

Nutritional Information

Serving Size: 1/6 recipe
Calories: 88
Sodium: 22 mg
Cholesterol: 0

Carbohydrate: 10 gm
Protein: 4 gm
Fat: 5 gm

Mixed Vegetable Side Dish

Anna Mary Beiler, Strasburg, Pennsylvania

I'm 12 years old and just love to cook. The first time I made this recipe for my family, everyone loved it. I'm sure you will, too!

1 cup sliced celery
1/2 cup chopped onion
2 garlic cloves, minced
3 tablespoons margarine
1 can (10-1/2 ounces) condensed low-sodium chicken broth
1/4 cup water
4 cups cubed peeled potatoes
1 cup julienned carrots
1/4 teaspoon pepper
1 tablespoon chopped fresh parsley

In a skillet, saute celery, onion and garlic in margarine until tender. Add the broth, water, potatoes, carrots and pepper. Bring to a boil; reduce heat. Cover and simmer 15-20 minutes or until potatoes are tender. Uncover and simmer for 5 minutes or until broth has slightly thickened, stirring occasionally. Sprinkle with parsley; serve immediately. **Yield:** 10 servings.

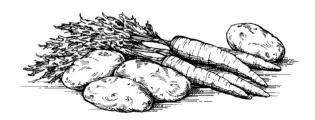

Exchanges: 1 Vegetable, 1/2 Starch, 1/2 Fat

Nutritional Information

Serving Size: 1/2 cup
Calories: 101
Sodium: 148 mg
Cholesterol: 2 mg

Carbohydrate: 15 gm
Protein: 2 gm
Fat: 4 gm

Carrot Pilaf

Grace Yaskovic, Branchville, New Jersey

Featuring shredded carrots and rice, this eye-catching recipe was the perfect addition to a "carrot patch" luncheon I once hosted.

1 cup shredded carrots
1/2 cup chopped onion
1 tablespoon margarine
1 cup uncooked long grain rice
1 can (14-1/2 ounces) low-sodium chicken broth
1 teaspoon lemon-pepper seasoning

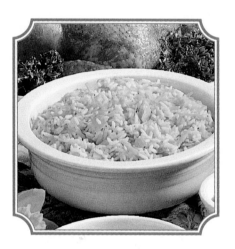

In a saucepan, saute carrots and onion in margarine until tender. Add rice and stir to coat. Stir in broth and lemon pepper; bring to a boil. Reduce heat; cover and simmer 20 minutes or until rice is tender. **Yield:** 6 servings.

Exchanges: 1-1/2 Starch, 1 Vegetable
Nutritional Information

Serving Size: 2/3 cup
Calories: 137
Sodium: 36 mg
Cholesterol: 0

Carbohydrate: 28 gm
Protein: 3 gm
Fat: 1 gm

Peas with Mushrooms

Mary Dennis, Bryan, Ohio

When I first saw this recipe calling for frozen peas, I have to admit I was skeptical. But not only is this side dish convenient, it's delicious!

1/2 pound fresh mushrooms, sliced
2 tablespoons sliced green onions
1 tablespoon margarine
1/4 teaspoon dried marjoram
1/8 teaspoon pepper
Dash ground nutmeg
1 package (10 ounces) frozen peas, cooked

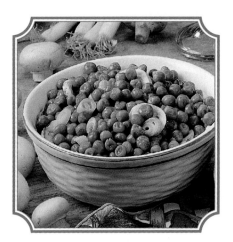

In a skillet over medium heat, saute the mushrooms and onions in margarine for 3-5 minutes. Add marjoram, pepper and nutmeg; mix well. Add peas and heat through. **Yield:** 4 servings.

Exchanges: 1 Vegetable, 1/2 Starch, 1/2 Fat

Nutritional Information

Serving Size: 1/4 recipe   Carbohydrate: 10 gm
Calories: 95   Protein: 4 gm
Sodium: 117 mg   Fat: 3 gm
Cholesterol: 0

Breads, Rolls & Muffins

Friends and family won't be able to resist the oven-fresh goodness of melt-in-your-mouth muffins, quick breads and yeast breads.

Cornmeal Muffins

Amelia Moody, Pasadena, Texas

In this part of the country, corn bread is often served with soup. These muffins are really easy to make, and they have good texture and flavor!

1 cup all-purpose flour
1 cup yellow cornmeal
1/3 cup sugar
1 tablespoon baking powder
1 teaspoon salt
2 tablespoons finely chopped onion
1 cup cream-style corn
1/2 cup light mayonnaise
3 tablespoons vegetable oil
Egg substitute equivalent to 1 egg

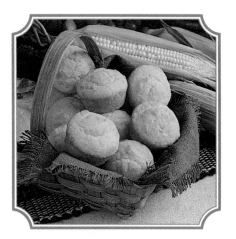

In a large mixing bowl, combine dry ingredients. Make a well in the center and add all remaining ingredients. Stir just until mixed. Spoon into 12 muffin cups coated with nonstick cooking spray. Bake at 400° for 20 minutes. **Yield:** 1 dozen.

Exchanges: 1-1/2 Starch, 1-1/2 Fat

Nutritional Information

Serving Size: 1 muffin
Calories: 189
Sodium: 434 mg
Cholesterol: 2 mg

Carbohydrate: 29 gm
Protein: 3 gm
Fat: 7 gm

Homemade Bread

Sandra Anderson, New York, New York

*We baked at least two batches of bread each week for our family of six...
and three never seemed to be enough! Everyone enjoyed this bread.*

2 packages (1/4 ounce *each*)
  active dry yeast
4-1/2 cups warm water (110° to 115°)
  6 tablespoons sugar
  2 tablespoons salt
  1/4 cup shortening, melted and
  cooled
  12 to 12-1/2 cups all-purpose
  flour

In a large mixing bowl, dissolve yeast in water. Add sugar, salt and shortening; stir until dissolved. Add half the flour; beat until smooth and the batter sheets with a spoon. Mix in enough remaining flour to form a soft dough that cleans the bowl. Turn onto a floured board. Knead 8-10 minutes or until smooth and elastic. Place in a bowl coated with nonstick cooking spray, turning once to grease top. Cover and allow to rise in a warm place until doubled, about 1-1/2 hours. Punch dough down. Cover and let rise again for 30 minutes. Divide dough into four parts and shape into loaves. Place in four 9-in. x 5-in. x 3-in. loaf pans coated with nonstick cooking spray. Cover and let rise in a warm place until doubled, about 30-45 minutes. Bake at 375° for 30-35 minutes or until golden brown. Remove from pans and allow to cool on wire racks. **Yield:** 4 loaves (16 slices each).

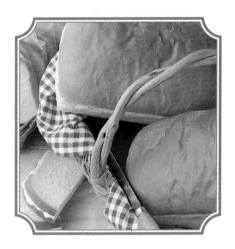

Exchanges: 1 Starch

Nutritional Information

Serving Size: 1 slice
Calories: 93
Sodium: 70 mg
Cholesterol: 0

Carbohydrate: 18 gm
Protein: 3 gm
Fat: 1 gm

Bran Muffins

Amber Sampson, Somonauk, Illinois

These hearty, nutritious muffins make a nice addition to all your meals no matter what time of day. They can bake while you prepare other menu items, so you can enjoy them hot from the oven.

1-1/4 cups all-purpose flour
1 tablespoon baking powder
1/3 cup sugar
1/2 teaspoon salt
1 cup 100% bran cereal
1 cup skim milk
1 egg
1/4 cup vegetable oil

Combine flour, baking powder, sugar and salt; set aside. In a mixing bowl, combine cereal and milk; let stand for 2 minutes. Add egg and oil; mix well. Add dry ingredients, stirring just until combined. Spoon into 12 muffin cups coated with nonstick cooking spray. Bake at 400° for 18-20 minutes or until golden brown. Serve warm. **Yield:** 1 dozen.

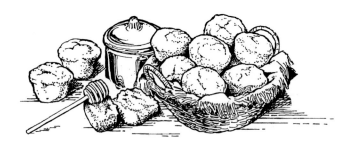

Exchanges: 1-1/2 Starch, 1/2 Fat
Nutritional Information

Serving Size: 1 muffin
Calories: 116
Sodium: 299 mg
Cholesterol: 18 mg

Carbohydrate: 23 gm
Protein: 4 gm
Fat: 2 gm

Zwieback Rolls

Martha Buhler, Dalles, Oregon

When Mother baked zwieback rolls—which means "twice baked"—she'd guard them, lest they disappear quickly! She would bake them on Sundays when friends came by for "fsapa", a meal of cold meat, cheese, jelly and coffee.

1 package (1/4 ounce) active dry yeast
1 teaspoon sugar
1/2 cup warm water (110° to 115°)
6 to 6-1/2 cups all-purpose flour
1 tablespoon salt
3/4 cup shortening, melted and cooled
2 cups warm skim milk (110° to 115°)

Dissolve yeast and sugar in water; set aside. In a large mixing bowl, combine 3 cups flour, salt, shortening, milk and yeast mixture. Beat well. Add enough of the remaining flour to form a soft dough. Turn onto a lightly floured board; knead until smooth and elastic, about 6-8 minutes. Dough should be soft. Place dough in a bowl coated with nonstick cooking spray; cover and allow to rise in a warm place until doubled, about 1 hour. Punch dough down and divide into four pieces. Divide three of the pieces into eight pieces each; shape into smooth balls and place on baking sheets coated with nonstick cooking spray. Divide remaining dough into 24 balls. Press 1 small ball atop each larger ball. Cover and let rise until doubled, about 45 minutes. Bake at 375° for 30 minutes or until golden. **Yield:** 2 dozen.

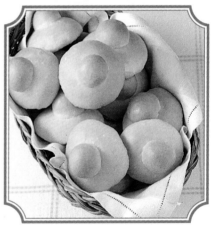

Exchanges: 2 Starch, 1 Fat

Nutritional Information

Serving Size: 1 roll
Calories: 186
Sodium: 299 mg
Cholesterol: 0

Carbohydrate: 27 gm
Protein: 4 gm
Fat: 6 gm

Pop-Up Bread

Bea Aubry, Dubuque, Iowa

One reason I like this bread is it's ready in such a short time. Plus, it always wins compliments. I've served it with homemade soup and fruit salads. It makes great sandwiches, too.

3 to 3-1/2 cups all-purpose flour
1 package (1/4 ounce) active dry yeast
1/2 cup milk
1/2 cup water
1/2 cup vegetable oil
1/4 cup sugar
1 teaspoon salt
2 eggs, beaten
1 cup (4 ounces) shredded cheddar cheese

Combine 1-1/2 cups flour and yeast. Heat milk, water, oil, sugar and salt until warm (120°-130°), stirring to blend; add to flour mixture along with eggs and cheese. Beat with an electric mixer or by hand until batter is smooth. Using a spoon, mix in the remaining flour (batter will be stiff). Divide batter and spoon into two 1-lb. coffee cans coated with nonstick cooking spray. Cover with plastic lids. Let rise in a warm place until batter is about 1/4 to 1/2 in. below plastic lids, about 45-60 minutes. Remove lids and bake at 375° for 30-35 minutes. Cool for 15 minutes in cans before removing. Cool on wire rack. **Yield:** 2 loaves (16 slices each).

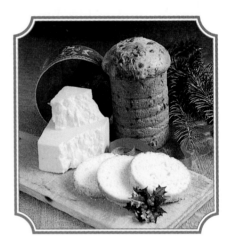

Exchanges: 1 Starch, 1 Fat
Nutritional Information

Serving Size: 1 slice
Calories: 111
Sodium: 98 mg
Cholesterol: 23 mg

Carbohydrate: 13 gm
Protein: 3 gm
Fat: 5 gm

Soft Breadsticks

Hazel Fritchie, Palestine, Illinois

My family never tires of these homemade breadsticks. As a matter of fact, I've been making them for 30 years! I think you'll agree they're better than any store-bought variety.

1 package (1/4 ounce) active dry yeast
1 cup warm water (110° to 115°)
3 tablespoons sugar
1 teaspoon salt
1/4 cup vegetable oil
3 cups all-purpose flour, *divided*
Cornmeal
1 egg white
1 tablespoon water

In a mixing bowl, dissolve yeast in water. Add sugar, salt and oil; stir until dissolved. Add 2 cups of flour; beat until smooth. Add enough remaining flour to form a soft dough. Turn onto a floured board; knead until smooth and elastic, about 6-8 minutes. Place in a bowl coated with nonstick cooking spray, turning once to grease top. Cover and let rise in a warm place until doubled, about 1 hour. Punch dough down and divide into 12 portions. Using your hands, roll each portion into a 10-in. x 1/2-in. strip. Place 1 in. apart on a baking sheet coated with nonstick cooking spray and sprinkled with cornmeal. Let rise, uncovered, until doubled, about 45-60 minutes. Beat egg white and water; brush over breadsticks. Place baking sheet on middle rack of oven; place a large shallow pan filled with boiling water on lowest rack. Bake at 400° for 10 minutes. Brush again with egg white. Bake 5 minutes more or until golden brown. **Yield:** 1 dozen.

Exchanges: 2 Starch, 1 Fat

Nutritional Information

Serving Size: 1 breadstick
Calories: 178
Sodium: 194 mg
Cholesterol: 0

Carbohydrate: 29 gm
Protein: 4 gm
Fat: 5 gm

Best Bran Muffins

Suzanne Smith, Framingham, Massachusetts

*Having these muffins for breakfast provides a good start to a busy day.
My husband loves pineapple, which makes these muffins moist...and delicious!*

1/2 cup rolled oats
1 cup all-purpose flour
1 cup whole wheat flour
1/2 cup all-bran cereal
1/2 teaspoon salt
1 teaspoon baking powder
1 teaspoon baking soda
1 egg, beaten
1/4 cup vegetable oil
1/2 cup molasses
3/4 cup buttermilk
1 can (8 ounces) crushed pineapple
   in natural juices, undrained
1/2 cup chopped nuts

In a mixing bowl, combine first seven ingredients. Make a well in the center. Combine the egg, oil, molasses, buttermilk and pineapple. Pour into well; mix until dry ingredients are moistened. Stir in nuts.

Coat 18 muffin cups with nonstick cooking spray; fill two-thirds full with batter. Bake at 400° for 12 minutes or until golden brown. **Yield:** 1-1/2 dozen.

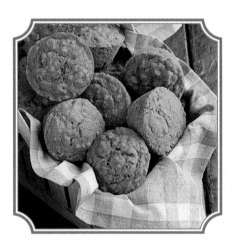

Exchanges: 1 Starch, 1 Fat, 1/2 Fruit
Nutritional Information

Serving Size: 1 muffin
Calories: 151
Sodium: 221 mg
Cholesterol: 16 mg

Carbohydrate: 22 gm
Protein: 4 gm
Fat: 6 gm

Braided Almond–Herb Bread

Ruth Peterson, Jenison, Michigan

My neighbor had just taken a loaf of this bread out of the oven when I stopped by. It was so fragrant and attractive that I just had to have the recipe!

**1 package (1/4 ounce) active dry
 yeast
2 tablespoons sugar
1/4 cup warm water (110° to 115°)
1/4 cup margarine
1 teaspoon salt
1 cup warm milk (110° to 115°)
3-1/2 to 4 cups all-purpose flour
1 teaspoon dried rosemary, crushed
1 teaspoon dill weed
1/2 teaspoon dried marjoram,
 crushed
1/2 cup finely chopped almonds,
 toasted,** *divided*
**1 egg, beaten
1 tablespoon water**

Dissolve yeast and sugar in warm water; set aside. In large mixing bowl, combine margarine, salt and milk. Stir in yeast mixture, 2 cups flour, herbs and 2 tablespoons almonds. Beat until well-mixed. Stir in enough remaining flour to form a soft dough. Turn onto a floured surface and knead until smooth and elastic, about 6-8 minutes. Place dough in a bowl coated with nonstick cooking spray, turning once to grease top. Cover; let rise in warm place until doubled, about 1 hour. Punch dough down and cut off a third; set aside. Divide remaining dough into three equal parts, shaping each into a 14-in. rope. Braid ropes and place on a baking sheet coated with nonstick cooking spray. Divide set-aside dough into three ropes and braid. Place smaller braid on top of larger braid. Cover; let rise until doubled, about 1 hour. Combine egg and water. Brush over entire loaf; sprinkle with remaining almonds. Bake at 375° for 30 minutes. **Yield:** 1 loaf.

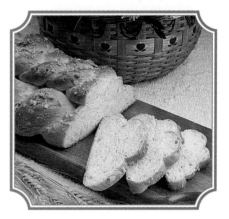

Exchanges: 1–1/4 Starch, 1 Fat
Nutritional Information
Serving Size: 1 slice
Calories: 130
Sodium: 148 mg
Cholesterol: 15 mg

Carbohydrate: 19 gm
Protein: 4 gm
Fat: 5 gm

Sugarless Fruit/Nut Muffins

Fern Albertson, Spokane, Washington

Once you've tasted these deliciously sweet, chewy gems, you'll be making them again and again. They freeze well, too, for a quick anytime snack!

1 cup chopped dates
1/2 cup raisins
1/2 cup chopped prunes
1 cup water
1/2 cup margarine, cut into pats
1/4 teaspoon salt
2 eggs, beaten
1 teaspoon vanilla extract
1 cup all-purpose flour
1 teaspoon baking soda
1/2 cup chopped nuts

In a saucepan, combine dates, raisins, prunes and water. Bring to a boil and boil for 5 minutes. Stir in margarine and salt. Set aside to cool. Add remaining ingredients; stir just until dry ingredients are moistened. Spoon into mini-muffin cups coated with nonstick cooking spray. Bake at 350° for 15 minutes. **Yield:** 32 mini-muffins.

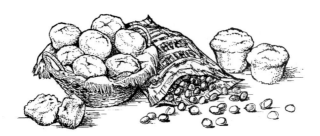

Exchanges: 1 Fat, 1/2 Fruit, 1/2 Starch
Nutritional Information
Serving Size: 1 muffin
Calories: 94
Sodium: 52 mg
Cholesterol: 14 mg

Carbohydrate: 12 gm
Protein: 2 gm
Fat: 4 gm

Italian Parmesan Bread

Frances Poste, Wall, South Dakota

When my grown children come home for visits, they always ask me to make this bread. It's also a hit whenever I take it to church socials and potluck suppers.

1 package (1/4 ounce) active dry
   yeast
1 cup warm water (110° to 115°)
3 cups all-purpose flour, *divided*
5 tablespoons margarine, softened,
   divided
1 egg, beaten
2 tablespoons sugar
1 teaspoon salt
1-1/2 teaspoons dried minced onion
1/2 teaspoon Italian seasoning
1/2 teaspoon garlic salt
1/2 cup grated Parmesan cheese,
   divided

In a mixing bowl, dissolve yeast in water. Add 2 cups flour, 4 tablespoons margarine, egg, sugar, salt and seasonings. Beat on low until mixed, about 30 seconds; increase speed to medium and continue beating for 2 minutes. Stir in remaining flour and 1/3 cup cheese; beat until smooth. Cover bowl and let rise in a warm place until doubled, about 1 hour. Stir batter 25 strokes. Spread into a 1-1/2-qt. casserole coated with nonstick cooking spray. Melt remaining margarine; brush over top. Sprinkle with remaining cheese. Cover and let rise until doubled, about 30 minutes. Bake at 350° for 35 minutes or until golden brown. Cool on wire rack 10 minutes before removing from the casserole. **Yield:** 1 loaf (16 slices).

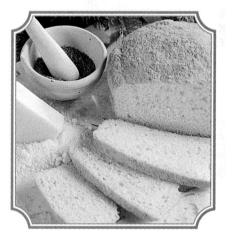

Exchanges: 1 Starch, 1/2 Fat

Nutritional Information

Serving Size: 1 slice
Calories: 97
Sodium: 216 mg
Cholesterol: 21 mg

Carbohydrate: 13 gm
Protein: 3 gm
Fat: 3 gm

No-Knead Honey Oatmeal Bread

Janice Dancer, Williamstown, Vermont

We especially enjoy this tasty bread because we feel using honey as a natural sweetener means healthier eating. We use the bread for both toast and sandwiches. It's great for special occasions...or, for that matter, anytime!

2 cups water, *divided*
1 cup rolled oats
1/3 cup margarine, softened
1/3 cup honey
1 tablespoon salt
2 packages (1/4 ounce *each***)
   active dry yeast**
1 egg
4 to 5 cups all-purpose flour

In a saucepan, heat 1 cup water to boiling. Stir in oats, margarine, honey and salt. Cool to lukewarm. Heat remaining water to 110°-115° and dissolve yeast. In a large mixing bowl, combine yeast mixture, egg, 2 cups flour and the oat mixture. Beat until the ingredients are combined and the batter is smooth. By hand, add enough remaining flour to make a stiff batter. Spread batter evenly into two 8-1/2-in. x 4-1/2-in. x 2-1/2-in. loaf pans coated with nonstick cooking spray. Smooth tops of loaves. Cover and let rise in a warm place until doubled, about 35-40 minutes. Bake at 375° for 40-45 minutes. Remove from pans to cool on wire racks. **Yield:** 2 loaves (16 slices each).

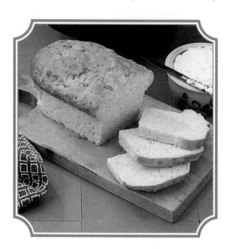

Exchanges: 1 Starch
Nutritional Information

Serving Size: 1 slice
Calories: 81
Sodium: 175 mg
Cholesterol: 6 mg

Carbohydrate: 14 gm
Protein: 2 gm
Fat: 2 gm

Cherry Blossom Muffins

Anna Mae Ackerman, Spearville, Kansas

Just because you have to curtail cholesterol doesn't mean you can't munch on a muffin! These moist muffins are bursting with pecans and cherry filling.

1/4 cup egg substitute
2/3 cup orange juice
2 tablespoons sugar
2 tablespoons vegetable oil
2 cups low-fat baking mix
1/2 cup chopped pecans
1/2 cup sugar-free cherry fruit spread

In a bowl, combine egg substitute, orange juice, sugar and oil. Add baking mix; stir for 30 seconds. Fold in pecans. Coat muffin cups with nonstick cooking spray or use paper liners; fill cups one-third full. Top each with 2 teaspoons fruit spread; cover with the remaining batter. Bake at 400° for 20-25 minutes or until muffins test done. Cool in pan 10 minutes before removing to a wire rack. **Yield:** 9 muffins.

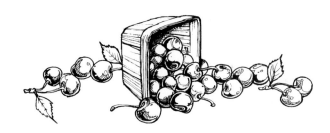

Exchanges: 2 Starch, 2 Fat

Nutritional Information

Serving Size: 1 muffin
Calories: 241
Sodium: 330 mg
Cholesterol: trace

Carbohydrate: 36 gm
Protein: 4 gm
Fat: 10 gm

Cinnamon Raisin Bread

Joan Hutter, Warnick, Rhode Island

My grandma's raisin bread is a long-standing tradition in our family.

2 packages (1/4 ounce *each*)
    active dry yeast
1/3 cup warm water (110° to 115°)
5-1/2 to 6 cups all-purpose flour
    1 cup warm milk (110° to 115°)
    2 eggs, lightly beaten
1/2 cup sugar
    6 tablespoons margarine, softened
1-1/4 teaspoons salt
FILLING:
1-1/3 cups golden raisins
1-1/3 cups dark raisins
    1 cup water
1/3 cup apple juice *or* cider
    1 tablespoon ground cinnamon
    1 egg, beaten

In a mixing bowl, dissolve yeast in water; let stand for 5 minutes. Add 2 cups flour, milk, eggs, sugar, margarine and salt. Beat on medium for 2 minutes. Add enough remaining flour to form a soft dough. Turn onto a floured board; knead until smooth and elastic, about 6-8 minutes. Place in a greased bowl, turning once to grease top. Cover and let rise in a warm place until doubled, about 1 hour. In a saucepan, bring first five filling ingredients to a boil. Reduce heat to medium; cook and stir for 15 minutes or until almost all the liquid is absorbed. Remove from heat; set aside. Punch dough down and knead 1 minute. Divide in half. Roll each half into a 12-in. x 8-in. rectangle; brush with egg. Spread half of filling over each rectangle to within 1/2 in. of edges. Roll up jelly roll fashion; pinch to seal. Place each loaf, seam side down, in a greased 9-in. x 5-in. x 3-in. loaf pan. Cover and let rise until doubled, about 1 hour. Cover loosely and bake at 350° for 35-40 minutes. **Yield:** 2 loaves (20 slices each).

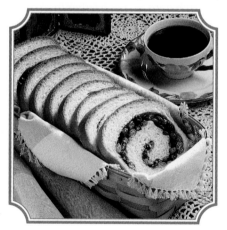

Exchanges: 1 Starch, 1 Fruit
Nutritional Information

Serving Size: 1 slice
Calories: 131
Sodium: 103 mg
Cholesterol: 11 mg

Carbohydrate: 25 gm
Protein: 3 gm
Fat: 2 gm

Freeze-and-Bake Rolls

Jayne Duce, Raymond, Alberta

Almost any occasion's right for these handy rolls—I keep them in the freezer for Sunday meals and for company (they have never failed to taste fresh).

**2 packages (1/4 ounce *each*)
   active dry yeast**
1-1/2 cups warm water (110° to 115°)
**1/2 cup plus 2 teaspoons sugar,
   *divided***
**1-1/2 cups warm skim milk (110° to
   115°)**
1/4 cup vegetable oil
4 teaspoons salt
7-1/2 to 8-1/2 cups all-purpose flour

In a large mixing bowl, dissolve yeast in water. Add 2 teaspoons sugar; let stand for 5 minutes. Add milk, oil, salt and remaining sugar. Add enough flour to form a stiff dough. Turn onto a floured surface; knead until smooth and elastic, about 6-8 minutes. Place in a bowl coated with nonstick cooking spray, turning once to grease top. Cover and let rise in a warm place until doubled, about 1-1/2 hours. Punch dough down. Divide into four pieces. Cover three pieces with plastic wrap. Divide one piece into 12 balls. To form knots, roll each ball into a 10-in. rope; tie into a knot and pinch ends together. Repeat with remaining dough. Place rolls on baking sheets coated with nonstick cooking spray; brush with melted butter. Cover and let rise until doubled, about 20-30 minutes. To serve immediately, bake at 375° for 15-18 minutes. To freeze for later use, partially bake at 300° for 15 minutes. Allow to cool; freeze. Reheat frozen rolls at 375° for 12-15 minutes or until browned. **Yield:** 4 dozen.

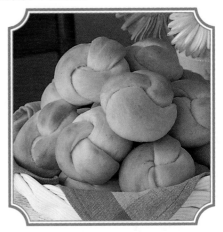

Exchanges: 1–1/2 Starch
Nutritional Information

Serving Size: 1 roll
Calories: 120
Sodium: 197 mg
Cholesterol: trace

Carbohydrate: 24 gm
Protein: 3 gm
Fat: 1 gm

White Casserole Bread

Lona Sage, Belvidere, Illinois

This bread won a blue ribbon when I entered it in a competition at a local fair. No matter how many times I prepare it, friends and family always proclaim it a winner!

1 package (1/4 ounce) active dry yeast
1-1/4 cups warm water (110° to 115°)
1 tablespoon sugar
1/2 teaspoon salt
2-1/2 to 3 cups all-purpose flour

In a large mixing bowl, dissolve yeast in water. Add sugar, salt and 1-1/2 cups flour; beat until smooth. Add enough remaining flour to form a soft dough. Turn onto a floured board; knead until smooth and elastic, about 6-8 minutes. Place in a bowl coated with nonstick cooking spray, turning once to grease top. Cover and let rise in a warm place until doubled, about 1 hour. Punch dough down. Shape into a round loaf and place in a 1-qt. baking dish coated with nonstick cooking spray. Cover and let rise until doubled, about 30 minutes. Using a sharp knife, make three slashes across the top. Bake at 350° for 40-45 minutes. Remove from dish to cool on a wire rack. **Yield:** 1 loaf (16 slices).

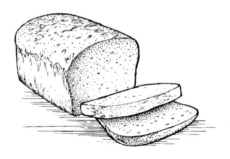

Exchanges: 1 Starch
Nutritional Information

Serving Size: 1 slice
Calories: 90
Sodium: 73 mg
Cholesterol: 0

Carbohydrate: 21 gm
Protein: 3 gm
Fat: trace

Honey Wheat Bread

Dorothy Anderson, Ottawa, Kansas

This recipe produces two beautiful loaves that have wonderful texture and slice well. The aroma of this bread baking can cut the chill from a cool autumn day.

2-1/2 to 3 cups all-purpose flour
3-1/2 cups whole wheat flour, *divided*
2 packages (1/4 ounce *each*)
  active dry yeast
1 cup skim milk
1-1/4 cups water
1/4 cup honey
3 tablespoons margarine
1 tablespoon salt

In a large mixing bowl, combine 2 cups all-purpose flour, 2 cups whole wheat flour and yeast. In a saucepan, heat milk, water, honey, margarine and salt to 120°-130°; add to flour mixture. Blend on low speed until moistened; beat on medium for 3 minutes. Gradually stir in remaining whole wheat flour and enough of the remaining all-purpose flour to form a soft dough. Turn onto a floured board; knead until smooth and elastic, about 6-8 minutes. Place in a bowl coated with nonstick cooking spray, turning once to grease top.

Cover and let rise in a warm place until doubled, about 1 hour. Punch dough down. Shape into two loaves; place in 8-in. x 4-in. x 2-in. loaf pans coated with nonstick cooking spray. Cover and let rise until doubled, about 1 hour. Bake at 375° for 40-45 minutes. Remove from pans to cool on wire racks. **Yield:** 2 loaves.

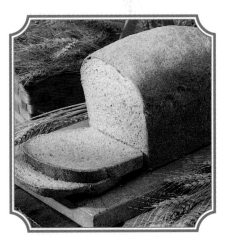

Exchanges: 1 Starch

Nutritional Information

Serving Size: One 1/2-inch slice
Calories: 99
Sodium: 216 mg
Cholesterol: 0

Carbohydrate: 19 gm
Protein: 3 gm
Fat: 1 gm

Golden Potato Rolls

Noni Ruegner, Salt Lake City, Utah

My mother nurtured my love for cooking when I was growing up.
Of course, Dad was always a willing taste-tester!

1 package (1/4 ounce) active dry
    yeast
1/2 cup warm water (110° to 115°)
1 cup skim milk
3/4 cup margarine
1-1/4 cups mashed potatoes (without
    added milk or margarine)
1/2 cup sugar
2 teaspoons salt
8 to 8-1/2 cups all-purpose flour
2 eggs, beaten

Dissolve yeast in water; set aside. In a saucepan, combine milk, margarine and potatoes; cook and stir over low heat just until margarine is melted. Remove from the heat and place in a large bowl with sugar, salt, 2 cups of flour and the yeast mixture. Add eggs; mix well. Cover loosely and allow to stand for 2 hours (the dough will be like a sponge). Stir in enough of the remaining flour to make a soft dough. Turn onto a floured surface and knead until smooth and elastic, about 6 minutes. Place in a bowl coated with nonstick cooking spray, turning once to grease top. Cover and let rise in a warm place until doubled, about 1 hour. Punch down and divide into thirds. On a floured surface, roll each portion into a 12-in. circle. Cut each circle into 12 pie-shaped wedges. Beginning at the wide end, roll up each wedge. Place rolls, point side down, 2 in. apart on baking sheets coated with nonstick cooking spray. Cover and let rise 30 minutes or until nearly doubled. Bake at 400° for 15 minutes or until golden. **Yield:** 3 dozen.

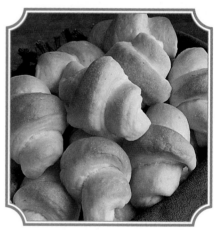

Exchanges: 1-1/2 Starch, 1 Fat
Nutritional Information

Serving Size: 1 roll
Calories: 170
Sodium: 168 mg
Cholesterol: 12 mg

Carbohydrate: 28 gm
Protein: 4 gm
Fat: 5 gm

Sweet Cornmeal Muffins

Marie Kramer, Kirkwood, Missouri

My husband was a big fan of the cornmeal muffins from a restaurant we visited. I finally found a recipe that makes similar muffins...now these are his favorites.

2 tablespoons sugar
4 teaspoons vegetable oil
Egg substitute equivalent to 1 egg
2 tablespoons skim milk
1/4 cup cornmeal
1/4 cup all-purpose flour
1/2 teaspoon baking powder
Pinch salt

In a bowl, combine sugar, oil, egg substitute and milk; mix well. In another bowl, combine dry ingredients; stir in sugar mixture just until moistened. Pour into four muffin cups that have been lined with papers or coated with nonstick cooking spray. Bake at 400° for 15-18 minutes or until lightly browned. **Yield:** 4 muffins.

STOP THE STICKS! To keep paper baking cups from clinging to muffins, coat the inside of the cups with nonstick cooking spray before filling.

Exchanges: 1-1/2 Starch, 1 Fat
Nutritional Information

Serving Size: 1 muffin
Calories: 153
Sodium: 87 mg
Cholesterol: trace

Carbohydrate: 20 gm
Protein: 4 gm
Fat: 6 gm

Herb Bread

Darlene Miller, Linn, Missouri

The ladies from our church have frequent bake sales, and this bread is always a hot item. It only takes one taste to understand why that's so!

3 cups whole wheat flour
5 to 5-1/2 cups all-purpose flour
2 packages (1/4 ounce *each*) active dry yeast
3 tablespoons sugar
1 tablespoon salt
1 teaspoon dried sage
1/2 teaspoon dried thyme
1/2 teaspoon dried marjoram
1 small onion, minced
3 tablespoons vegetable oil
3 cups warm water (120° to 130°)
1 tablespoon skim milk
2 tablespoons grated Parmesan cheese

In a large mixing bowl, combine whole wheat flour, 1 cup all-purpose flour, yeast, sugar, salt, herbs, onion, oil and water. Beat with an electric mixer on low until moistened, then beat for 3 minutes at medium. By hand, stir in enough of the remaining flour to form a stiff dough. Place in a bowl coated with nonstick cooking spray, turning once to grease top. Cover and allow to rise until doubled, about 1 hour. Punch dough down. Shape into two balls and place in two 2-qt. casseroles coated with nonstick cooking spray. Cover and let rise until almost doubled, about 45 minutes. Brush tops with milk and sprinkle with Parmesan cheese. Bake at 350° for 40-45 minutes. Remove from casseroles to cool on a wire rack. **Yield:** 2 loaves (20 slices each).

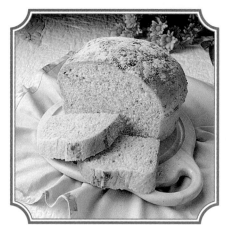

Exchanges: 1-1/4 Starch

Nutritional Information

Serving Size: 1 slice
Calories: 99
Sodium: 63 mg
Cholesterol: trace

Carbohydrate: 21 gm
Protein: 3 gm
Fat: trace

Honey-Wheat Sunflower Bread

Lillian Wittler, Wayne, Nebraska

This bread is both delicious and nutritious, and the sunflower seeds add a nice texture.

2 cups water (120° to 130°)
2-3/4 to 3-1/4 cups all-purpose *or* bread flour
2 packages (1/4 ounce *each*) active dry yeast
1 tablespoon sugar
2 cups whole wheat flour
1 cup old-fashioned oats
1/3 cup instant dry milk powder
1/4 cup margarine, melted and cooled
1/4 cup honey
2 teaspoons salt
1 cup unsalted sunflower seeds

In a mixing bowl, combine the water, 2 cups all-purpose or bread flour, yeast and sugar. Beat on low speed for 3 minutes. Cover and let rise in a warm place until doubled, about 30 minutes. (Mixture will be spongy.) Stir in whole wheat flour, oats, milk powder, margarine, honey and salt; mix well. Stir in sunflower seeds and enough of the remaining all-purpose or bread flour. Turn onto a lightly floured surface and knead until smooth and elastic, about 6-8 minutes. Shape into a ball. Place in a bowl coated with nonstick cooking spray, turning once to grease top. Cover and let rise until doubled, about 30-45 minutes. Punch down and divide in half. Cover and let rest 10 minutes. Shape into two loaves; place in two 8-in. x 4-in. x 2-in. loaf pans coated with nonstick cooking spray. Cover and let rise until doubled, about 30 minutes. Bake at 375° for 20 minutes. Cover with foil; bake 15 minutes longer. Remove from pans and cool on wire racks. **Yield:** 2 loaves (16 slices each).

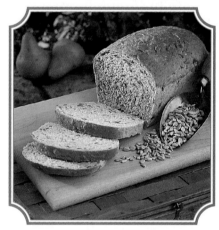

Exchanges: 1 Fat, 1 Starch

Nutritional Information

Serving Size: 1 slice
Calories: 121
Sodium: 162 mg
Cholesterol: trace

Carbohydrate: 18 gm
Protein: 4 gm
Fat: 4 gm

Apricot Walnut Bread

Diane Hixon, Niceville, Florida

Orange juice and oat bran add flavor and texture to this quick bread. My family enjoys it a lot for brekfast or snacking so I tend to keep the ingredients for this recipe on hand.

4 egg whites
2/3 cup water
1/2 cup orange juice
1/4 cup vegetable oil
1 teaspoon vanilla extract
3/4 cup uncooked oat bran hot cereal
1/2 cup chopped dried apricots
1-1/4 cups all-purpose flour
1/2 cup packed brown sugar
1 teaspoon baking powder
1/2 teaspoon baking soda
1/4 cup chopped walnuts

In a bowl, combine the first five ingredients. Stir in cereal and apricots. Combine flour, brown sugar, baking powder and soda; stir into apricot mixture just until moistened. Fold in nuts. Pour into a 8-in. x 4-in. x 2-in. loaf pan coated with nonstick cooking spray. Bake at 350° for 50-55 minutes or until bread tests done. Cool in pan 10 minutes; remove to wire rack. **Yield:** 1 loaf (16 slices).

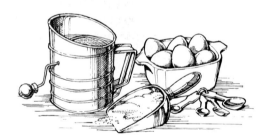

Exchanges: 1 Starch, 1 Fat, 1/2 Fruit

Nutritional Information

Serving Size: 1 slice
Calories: 141
Sodium: 42 mg
Cholesterol: 0

Carbohydrate: 20 gm
Protein: 4 gm
Fat: 5 gm

Chive Garden Rolls

Joanie Elbourn, Gardner, Massachusetts
(ALSO PICTURED ON FRONT COVER)

Everyone who's ever tried these rolls has found them hard to resist. They go especially well with a green salad or steaming bowl of soup.

1 egg
1 cup (8 ounces) fat-free cottage
   cheese
1/4 cup vegetable oil
2 teaspoons honey
1 teaspoon salt
1 package (1/4 ounce) active dry
   yeast
1/2 cup warm water (110° to 115°)
1/4 cup wheat germ
2-3/4 to 3-1/4 cups all-purpose flour
   3 tablespoons chopped fresh *or*
   dried chives
TOPPING:
   1 egg, beaten
   1 small onion, finely chopped

In a mixing bowl, combine the egg, cottage cheese, oil, honey and salt. Dissolve yeast in warm water; add to egg mixture. Add wheat germ and 1-1/2 cups flour. Mix on medium speed for 3 minutes. Add chives and enough remaining flour to form a soft dough. Turn onto a floured board; knead until smooth and elastic, about 10 minutes. Place in a bowl coated with non-stick cooking spray, turning once to grease top. Cover and let rise in a warm place until doubled, about 1 hour. Punch dough down; roll out to 3/4-in. thickness. Cut with a 3-in. round cutter. Place on baking sheets coated with nonstick cooking spray. Cover and let rise until doubled, about 45 minutes. Brush tops with egg and sprinkle with onion. Bake at 350° for 15-20 minutes or until golden brown. **Yield:** 1 dozen.

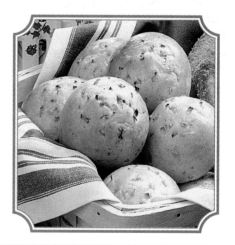

Exchanges: 2 Starch, 1 Fat

Nutritional Information

Serving Size: 1 roll
Calories: 205
Sodium: 270 mg
Cholesterol: 35 mg

Carbohydrate: 29 gm
Protein: 8 gm
Fat: 6 gm

Italian Bread

Virginia Slater, West Sunbury, Pennsylvania

You could say this recipe has stood the test of time. My mother–in–law taught me how to make this bread...now the recipe's been passed down to my daughter and two granddaughters.

2 packages (1/4 ounce *each*) active dry yeast
3 tablespoons sugar
3 tablespoons shortening
3 cups warm water (110° to 115°)
8 to 10 cups all-purpose flour
1 tablespoon salt
1 egg, beaten

Dissolve yeast, sugar and shortening in water. Stir in 4 cups flour, salt and egg; beat until smooth. Stir in enough remaining flour to form a stiff dough. Turn out onto a floured surface; knead until smooth and elastic, about 6-8 minutes. Place in a bowl coated with nonstick cooking spray, turning once to grease top. Cover and allow to rise in a warm place, punching dough down every 10 minutes, for 1 hour. Then allow dough to rise for 1 additional hour, or until doubled. Punch dough down; let rest 10 minutes. Divide into two loaves. Slash tops and place on baking pans or in two 9-in. x 5-in. x 3-in. loaf pans coated with nonstick cooking spray. Cover and let rise until doubled, about 1 hour. Bake at 350° for about 45 minutes or until golden brown. Remove from pans; cool on wire racks. **Yield:** 2 loaves.

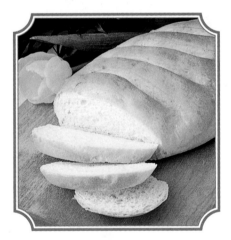

Exchanges: 1 Starch
Nutritional Information

Serving Size: One 1/2-inch slice
Calories: 94
Sodium: 130 mg
Cholesterol: 4 mg

Carbohydrate: 18 gm
Protein: 3 gm
Fat: 1 gm

Caraway Rye Bread

Connie Moore, Medway, Ohio

My family loves rye bread with its savory, nutty flavor. So one day, I decided to make it from scratch. Needless to say, the loaf disappeared in a hurry!

2 packages (1/4 ounce *each*) active dry yeast
1-1/2 cups warm water (110° to 115°), *divided*
3 tablespoons molasses
3 tablespoons margarine, melted
1 tablespoon caraway seed
1 teaspoon salt
1-1/2 to 2 cups all-purpose flour
1-1/2 cups whole wheat flour
1 cup rye flour

In mixing bowl, dissolve yeast in 1/2 cup water. Add molasses, margarine, caraway, salt and remaining water; mix well. Combine flours; add 3 cups to batter. Beat until smooth. Add enough remaining flour to form a firm dough. Turn onto a floured board; knead until smooth and elastic, 6-8 minutes. Place in a bowl coated with nonstick cooking spray, turning once to grease top. Cover and let rise in a warm place until doubled, about 1 hour. Punch dough down; shape into a round loaf. Place on a baking sheet coated with non-stick cooking spray. Cover and let rise until doubled, about 30 minutes. Bake at 375° for 20-25 minutes or until golden brown. **Yield:** 1 loaf (16 slices).

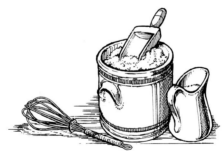

Exchanges: 2 Starch
Nutritional Information

Serving Size: 1 slice
Calories: 128
Sodium: 153 mg
Cholesterol: 0

Carbohydrate: 26 gm
Protein: 4 gm
Fat: 1 gm

Mini White Breads

Nila Towler, Baird, Texas

*These small, light loaves have wonderful flavor and texture.
I've found them to be the perfect size when cooking for a
smaller number or when preparing them for gifts around the holidays.*

1 package (1/4 ounce) active dry yeast
1 tablespoon sugar
1/3 cup warm water (110° to 115°)
2-1/4 to 2-1/2 cups all-purpose flour
1 teaspoon salt
1/2 cup milk
2 teaspoons margarine, melted

Combine yeast, sugar and water in a large mixing bowl. Add 1-1/2 cups of flour, salt, milk and margarine. Mix for 3 minutes on medium speed. Add enough remaining flour to form a soft dough. Turn onto a floured board; knead until smooth and elastic, 6-8 minutes. Place in a bowl coated with nonstick cooking spray, turning once to grease top. Cover and let rise in a warm place until doubled, about 45 minutes. Punch dough down. Divide in half; shape into two loaves and place in 5-3/4- in. x 3-1/8-in. x 2-1/4-in. pans coated with nonstick cooking spray. Cover and let rise until doubled, about 30 minutes. Bake at 375° for 30 minutes or until golden brown. Remove from pans; cool on wire racks. **Yield:** 2 mini loaves.

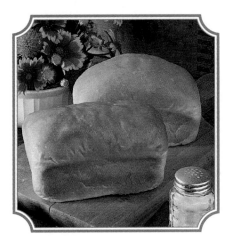

Exchanges: 1 Starch

Nutritional Information

Serving Size: One 1/2-inch slice
Calories: 69
Sodium: 135 mg
Cholesterol: 0

Carbohydrate: 14 gm
Protein: 2 gm
Fat: 1 gm

Sweet Treats

*From cakes, cookies and bars to ice cream,
pudding and pies, these delicious desserts will
satisfy any sweet tooth in a hurry.*

Strawberry Shortcake

Sue Gronholz, Columbus, Wisconsin

It seems I can never get enough of Grandma's shortcake! This recipe is special to me…it's the first thing I bake when my strawberries ripen in spring.

2 cups all-purpose flour
2 tablespoons sugar
4 teaspoons baking powder
1/2 teaspoon salt
1/2 teaspoon cream of tartar
1/2 cup margarine, softened
1 egg, beaten
2/3 cup skim milk
2 pints strawberries, sliced
Light whipped topping, optional

In a bowl, combine flour, sugar, baking powder, salt and cream of tartar. Cut in margarine until mixture forms coarse crumbs. Add the egg and milk; mix well. Spread into an 8-in. square baking pan coated with nonstick cooking spray. Bake at 375° for 20-25 minutes. Cut into squares; top with strawberries and whipped cream if desired. **Yield:** 9 servings.

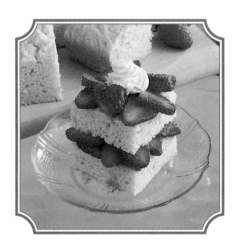

Exchanges: 2 Fat, 1-3/4 Starch
Nutritional Information

Serving Size: 1/9 recipe
Calories: 217
Sodium: 436 mg
Cholesterol: 24 mg

Carbohydrate: 27 gm
Protein: 5 gm
Fat: 11 gm
(Calculated without whipped topping)

Light 'n' Rich Chocolate Pudding

Andrea Chen, Binghamton, New York

Even those who strictly limit the sugar in their diet can dig in and enjoy a creamy chocolate pudding—thanks to this imaginative recipe I've found!

Artificial sweetener equivalent to 6 tablespoons sugar
   3 tablespoons baking cocoa
   3 tablespoons cornstarch
   2 cups skim milk
   1 teaspoon vanilla extract

In a saucepan, combine sweetener, cocoa and cornstarch. Whisk in the milk. Simmer, stirring constantly, until thickened, about 5 minutes. Stir in the vanilla. Cool. **Yield:** 4 servings.

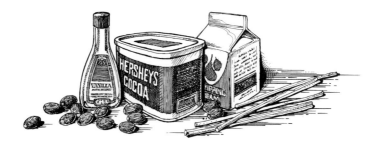

Exchanges: 3/4 Starch, 1/2 Milk

Nutritional Information

Serving Size: 1/4 recipe
Calories: 95
Sodium: 63 mg
Cholesterol: 2 mg

Carbohydrate: 17 gm
Protein: 5 gm
Fat: 1 gm

Sugarless Spice Cake

Jewell Curry, Albany, Oregon

This cake is perfect for folks who are watching their diet. It's easy to make and delicious!

2 cups raisins
2 cups water
1 cup unsweetened applesauce
2 eggs, beaten
2 tablespoons liquid artificial sweetener
3/4 cup vegetable oil
1 teaspoon baking soda
2 cups all-purpose flour
1-1/2 teaspoons ground cinnamon
1/2 teaspoon ground nutmeg
1 teaspoon vanilla extract
Light whipped topping, optional

In a saucepan, cook raisins in water until water evaporates. Add applesauce, eggs, sweetener and oil; mix well. Blend in baking soda and flour. Stir in cinnamon, nutmeg and vanilla. Pour into an 8-in. square baking pan coated with nonstick cooking spray. Bake at 350° for 25 minutes or until cake tests done. Garnish with whipped topping if desired. **Yield: 20 servings.**

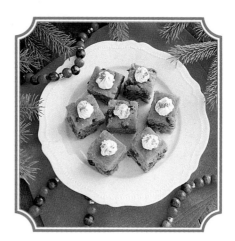

Exchanges: 2 Fat, 1 Starch, 1/2 Fruit

Nutritional Information

Serving Size: 1 piece
Calories: 181
Sodium: 18 mg
Cholesterol: 10 mg

Carbohydrate: 24 gm
Protein: 3 gm
Fat: 9 gm
(Calculated without whipped topping)

Orange-Date Bars

Sue Yaeger, Brookings, South Dakota

If you're looking to serve a lighter, more nutritious dessert, you'll appreciate this recipe. It's an appealing old-fashioned dessert that's full-flavored.

1 cup chopped dates
1/3 cup sugar
1/3 cup vegetable oil
1/2 cup orange juice
1 egg, beaten
1 cup all-purpose flour
1-1/2 teaspoons baking powder
1 tablespoon grated orange peel
1/2 cup chopped pecans

In a saucepan, combine dates, sugar, oil and juice. Cook for 5 minutes to soften dates. Cool. Add egg; mix well. Combine all remaining ingredients and stir into date mixture. Spread into an 8-in. square baking pan coated with nonstick cooking spray. Bake at 350° for 25-30 minutes. Cool before cutting. **Yield:** 3 dozen.

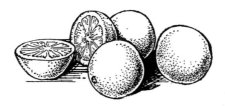

Exchanges: 1/2 Starch, 1/2 Fat

Nutritional Information

Serving Size: 1 bar
Calories: 56
Sodium: 12 mg
Cholesterol: 8 mg

Carbohydrate: 6 gm
Protein: 1 gm
Fat: 3 gm

Angel Food Cake

Sharon Voth, Alexander, Manitoba

*After just one taste, you'll agree this cake is heavenly!
I like to make it for special occasions throughout the year.*

1 cup cake flour
1-1/2 cups sugar, *divided*
2 cups egg whites (about 15 large eggs)
1-1/4 teaspoons cream of tartar
1 teaspoon vanilla extract
1/4 teaspoon almond extract
1/4 teaspoon salt

Sift flour and 1/2 cup sugar together four times; set aside. In a mixing bowl, combine egg whites, cream of tartar, extracts and salt; beat on high until soft peaks form but mixture is still moist and glossy. Add remaining sugar, 1/4 cup at a time, beating well after each addition. Sift flour mixture, a fourth at a time, over the egg white mixture; fold in gently, using about 15 strokes for each addition. Spoon batter into an ungreased 10-in. tube pan (pan will be very full). Bake at 375° for 35-40 minutes or until top crust is golden brown and cracks feel dry. Immediately invert cake in pan to cool completely. Loosen sides of cake from pan and remove. **Yield:** 16 servings.

A SMALL FUNNEL is handy for separating egg whites from egg yolks. Crack the egg over the funnel. The whites will run through, and the yolks will remain.

Exchanges: 1-1/2 Starch
Nutritional Information

Serving Size: 1 piece
Calories: 101
Sodium: 106 mg
Cholesterol: 0

Carbohydrate: 24 gm
Protein: 2 gm
Fat: trace

Special Chocolate Ice Cream

Alice Taylor, Swansboro, North Carolina

Being diabetic, I've learned to satisfy my sweet tooth with a number of different desserts. This ice cream is low in sugar—but you wouldn't know it by its smooth texture and delicious taste.

1 package (1.5 ounces) sugar-free instant chocolate pudding mix
6 packets artificial sweetener (equivalent to 1/4 cup sugar)
2 tablespoons baking cocoa
4 cups evaporated skim milk
1 teaspoon vanilla extract
4 ounces light frozen whipped topping, thawed

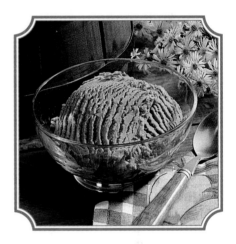

In a blender, combine the pudding mix, sweetener, cocoa, milk and vanilla; process on low until smooth. Fold in the whipped topping until smooth. Pour into a shallow 2-qt. freezer container. Cover and freeze for 30 minutes. Stir with a wire whisk; return to freezer until ready to serve. **Yield:** 12 servings.

Exchanges: 1 Skim Milk, 1/2 Starch, 1/2 Fat
Nutritional Information

Serving Size: 1/2 cup
Calories: 140
Sodium: 257 mg
Cholesterol: 4 mg

Carbohydrate: 20 gm
Protein: 10 gm
Fat: 3 gm

Apple Cobbler

Erlene Cornelius, Spring City, Texas

My daughter-in-law is a diabetic, so I came up with this recipe especially for her. But this cobbler is so good, the whole family enjoys it!

4 cups sliced peeled apples (about 3 large)
3/4 cup water, *divided*
1 tablespoon lemon juice
Pinch salt
1 tablespoon cornstarch
Artificial sweetener equivalent to 2 tablespoons sugar
1/2 teaspoon ground cinnamon
TOPPING:
1/2 cup all-purpose flour
1/2 teaspoon baking powder
1/4 teaspoon salt
4 teaspoons shortening
5 tablespoons skim milk

Put the apples, 1/2 cup water, lemon juice and salt in a microwave-safe 8-in. x 4-in. x 2-in. loaf pan. Microwave on high for 3 minutes. Stir, then cook 3 minutes more. Combine the cornstarch, sweetener cinnamon and remaining water; stir into hot apples. Microwave for 1 minute. For topping, combine flour, baking powder and salt in a bowl. Cut in shortening until mixture forms small crumbs. Stir in milk with a fork. Drop by heaping teaspoonfuls onto hot apple mixture. Bake at 400° for 20-25 minutes. **Yield:** 4 servings. **Editor's Note:** This recipe was tested in a 700-watt microwave oven. Use an artificial sweetener recommended for baking, such as Sweet 'N Low or Sweet One.

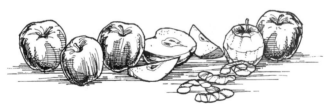

Exchanges: 1 Starch, 1 Fruit, 1 Fat
Nutritional Information

Serving Size: 1/4 recipe
Calories: 180
Sodium: 216 mg
Cholesterol: 0

Carbohydrate: 35 gm
Protein: 3 gm
Fat: 5 gm

Butterscotch Pumpkin Pie

Elizabeth Fehr, Cecil Lake, British Columbia

*When I'm in the mood for something sweet, this is the recipe
I reach for. The addition of butterscotch pudding makes this
a tasty twist on traditional pumpkin pie.*

1 cup graham cracker crumbs
1/4 cup margarine, melted
FILLING:
  1 package (.9 ounce) sugar-free
  instant butterscotch pudding mix
  1 cup skim milk
  1 cup cooked pumpkin
  1 teaspoon ground cinnamon
  1/2 teaspoon ground nutmeg
TOPPING:
  1 cup light whipped topping
  1 teaspoon vanilla extract

To make pie crust, combine crumbs and margarine; pat into a 9-in. pie plate. Bake at 350° for 10 minutes; cool. For filling, combine pudding mix and milk in a mixing bowl; beat well. Add pumpkin, cinnamon and nutmeg; mix well. Pour into crust. Chill for at least 2 hours. Combine topping ingredients; dollop on individual slices. **Yield:** 8 servings.

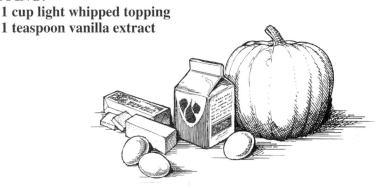

Exchanges: 2-1/2 Fat, 1 Starch
Nutritional Information
Serving Size: 1 slice with 2
tablespoons topping
Calories: 148
Sodium: 203 mg

Cholesterol: 1 mg
Carbohydrate: 17 gm
Protein: 3 gm
Fat: 9 gm

California Fresh Fruit Dip

Nancy Cutright, San Jose, California

I tried this dip at a potluck lunch and loved it. I think it represents my region of the country because of the abundance of fresh fruit grown here. My family especially enjoys it as a refreshing snack on hot summer afternoons.

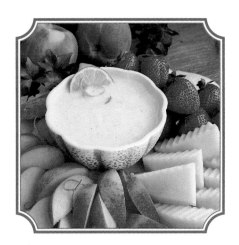

1 cup plain low-fat yogurt
2 tablespoons honey
2 tablespoons lime juice
1 teaspoon grated lime peel
1/4 teaspoon ground ginger

In a small bowl, combine all ingredients. Serve with fresh fruit. Cover and refrigerate leftovers. **Yield:** about 1 cup.

Exchanges: 1/4 Fruit, 1/4 Skim Milk

Nutritional Information

Serving Size: 2 tablespoons
Calories: 33
Sodium: 22 mg
Cholesterol: 1 mg

Carbohydrate: 7 gm
Protein: 2 gm
Fat: trace

Sugar-Free Raisin Bars

Betty Ruenholl, Syracuse, Nebraska

My mother is diabetic, so I keep these moist, golden bars on hand for dessert. I even serve them during the holidays. They're a nice light snack for everyone.

1 cup raisins
1/2 cup water
1/4 cup margarine
1 teaspoon ground cinnamon
1/4 teaspoon ground nutmeg
1 cup all-purpose flour
1 egg, lightly beaten
3/4 cup unsweetened applesauce
Artificial sweetener equivalent to 1
tablespoon sugar
1 teaspoon baking soda
1/4 teaspoon vanilla extract

In a saucepan over medium heat, cook raisins, water, margarine, cinnamon and nutmeg until margarine is melted; continue cooking for 3 minutes. Add all remaining ingredients. Spread into an 8-in. square baking dish coated with nonstick cooking spray. Bake at 350° for 25-30 minutes or until lightly browned. **Yield:** 16 bars. **Editor's Note:** Use an artificial sweetener recommended for baking, such as Sweet 'N Low or Sweet One.

Exchanges: 1 Starch, 1/2 Fat
Nutritional Information

Serving Size: 1 bar
Calories: 92
Sodium: 97 mg
Cholesterol: 13 mg

Carbohydrate: 15 gm
Protein: 2 gm
Fat: 3 gm

Angel Food Ice Cream Cake

Madelon Howland, Sterling, New York

I made this cake for my grandson's birthday and it was a hit—the children loved the ice cream inside. It looks as good as it tastes!

1 angel food cake (8 inches)
1/2 gallon sugar-free vanilla ice cream, slightly softened
2 quarts fresh strawberries
Sugar substitute to taste, optional

Cut the cake in half; tear one half into small pieces and set aside. Cut the other half into 12-14 thin slices; arrange in the bottom of a waxed paper-lined 13-in. x 9-in. x 2-in. baking pan, overlapping as needed. Spread softened ice cream over cake, pressing down to smooth. Gently press the small cake pieces into ice cream. Cover and freeze. Just before serving, slice strawberries and sweeten to taste if desired. Cut dessert into squares and top with strawberries. **Yield:** 15 servings.

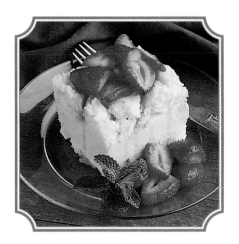

Exchanges: 1-1/2 Starch, 1 Fat, 1/2 Fruit

Nutritional Information

Serving Size: 1/15 recipe
Calories: 183
Sodium: 131 mg
Cholesterol: 15 mg

Carbohydrate: 34 gm
Protein: 6 gm
Fat: 4 gm

'Mock' Sour Cream Raisin Pie

Danile Keily-Zent, Yakima, Washington

This old-fashioned dessert really is easy-as-pie to prepare. It's perfect for entertaining because it can be made ahead of time.

1 cup skim milk
1 cup (8 ounces) plain yogurt
1 package (.8 ounce) sugar-free cook-and-serve vanilla pudding mix
1/2 teaspoon ground allspice
3/4 cup raisins
1 pastry shell (9 inches), baked

In a saucepan, combine milk and yogurt. Add the pudding mix; cook and stir constantly until mixture boils and thickens. Stir in allspice. Add raisins; mix well. Let cool for 10 minutes, stirring occasionally. Pour into pastry shell. Chill at least 2 hours. **Yield:** 8 servings.

> **STOP SHELL SHRINKAGE!** To prevent your pie shell from shrinking as it bakes, put rolled pastry in a pie plate, then place an empty pie plate inside it. Bake 10 minutes. Remove the empty plate; continue baking until crust is brown.

Exchanges: 1-1/2 Fat, 1 Fruit, 1/2 Skim Milk

Nutritional Information

Serving Size: 1 slice
Calories: 175
Sodium: 210 mg
Cholesterol: 1 mg

Carbohydrate: 24 gm
Protein: 4 gm
Fat: 8 gm

Yogurt Parfait

Dottye Wolf, Rolla, Missouri

*I'm on a restricted diet, but my husband is not. So, I'll
often make two different single-serving recipes. Besides being
a great dessert, this is a delicious breakfast or luncheon treat.*

1 carton (6 ounces) low-fat, sugar-
 free yogurt (any flavor)
1/4 cup low-fat granola
1/2 cup sliced fresh fruit (apple,
 strawberries, banana, etc.)

In a parfait glass or large glass mug, layer one-third of the yogurt, half of the
granola and then half of the fruit. Repeat
layers. Top with the remaining yogurt.
Yield: 1 serving.

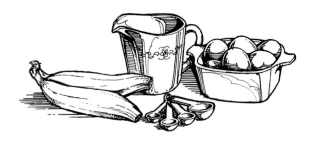

Exchanges: 1 Skim Milk, 1 Fat, 1/2 Starch, 1/2 Fruit
Nutritional Information

Serving Size: 1 recipe
Calories: 209
Sodium: 171 mg
Cholesterol: 3 mg

Carbohydrate: 30 gm
Protein: 10 gm
Fat: 5 gm

Sugarless Apple Cookies

Martha Gradeless, Garrett, Indiana

*When I found out I was diabetic, I began looking for more suitable recipes.
These soft, chewy cookies are so moist and delicious, you'll never miss the sugar.*

3/4 cup chopped dates
1/2 cup finely chopped peeled
apple
1/2 cup raisins
1/2 cup water
1 cup plus 1 tablespoon
all-purpose flour
1 teaspoon ground cinnamon
1 teaspoon baking soda
2 eggs
1 teaspoon liquid artificial
sweetener

In a large saucepan, combine dates, apple,
raisins and water. Bring to a boil; reduce
heat and simmer for 3 minutes. Remove
from the heat; cool. Combine flour, cinnamon and baking soda. Stir into apple
mixture and mix well. Combine eggs
and sweetener; add to batter. Drop by tablespoonfuls onto a nonstick baking
sheet. Bake at 350° for 10-12 minutes.
Yield: 2 dozen.

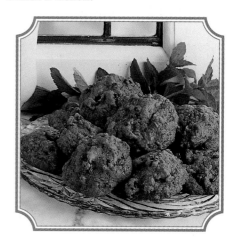

Exchanges: 1/2 Starch, 1/2 Fruit
Nutritional Information

Serving Size: 1 cookie
Calories: 54
Sodium: 24 mg
Cholesterol: 18 mg

Carbohydrate: 11 gm
Protein: 1 gm
Fat: 1 gm

Raspberry Crunch Brownies

Rita Winterberger, Huson, Montana

These rich brownies with dark chocolate flavor and nut–like crunch prove that desserts don't have to be full of fat to be splendid.

1/4 cup vegetable oil
1-1/4 cups sugar
4 egg whites
1 cup all-purpose flour
1/2 teaspoon baking powder
1/4 teaspoon salt
2/3 cup baking cocoa
1-1/2 teaspoons vanilla extract
1/4 cup raspberry jam
2 tablespoons Grape-Nuts cereal

In a mixing bowl, beat oil and sugar. Add egg whites and continue beating until well mixed. Combine flour, baking powder, salt and cocoa; add to egg white mixture and beat until moistened. Stir in vanilla. Batter will be thick. Spread batter into a 9-in. square baking pan with nonstick cooking spray. Bake at 350° for 20-25 minutes or until a toothpick inserted in the center comes out clean. Cool 10 minutes on a wire rack. Spread with jam and sprinkle with Grape-Nuts. Cool completely. **Yield:** 2 dozen.

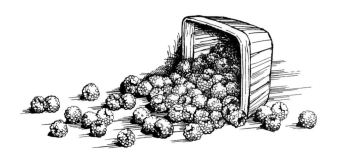

Exchanges: 1 Starch, 1/2 Fat
Nutritional Information

Serving Size: 1 brownie
Calories: 105
Sodium: 47 mg
Cholesterol: 0

Carbohydrate: 19 gm
Protein: 2 gm
Fat: 3 gm

Old-Fashioned Bread Pudding

Wynona Strietelmeier, Indianapolis, Indiana

Through the years, I've made this bread pudding quite often and am asked for the recipe each time. I think folks find this dessert so appealing because of its comforting taste and texture.

2 cups skim milk
1/2 cup egg substitute
1 teaspoon vanilla extract
Artificial sweetener equivalent to 1 teaspoon sugar
4 slices stale bread, cut into 1-inch cubes
2 tablespoons raisins
1/2 teaspoon ground cinnamon

Combine milk, egg substitute, vanilla and sweetener in a bowl. Add bread cubes and raisins; stir gently. Pour into a 1-qt. baking dish coated with nonstick cooking spray. Sprinkle with cinnamon. Place in a shallow pan; add 1 in. of water. Bake at 350° for 50 minutes or until a knife inserted near the center comes out clean. **Yield:** 6 servings. **Editor's Note:** Use an artificial sweetener recommended for baking, such as Sweet 'N Low or Sweet One.

Exchanges: 1 Starch, 1/2 Meat

Nutritional Information

Serving Size: 1/6 recipe
Calories: 113
Sodium: 165 mg
Cholesterol: 1 mg

Carbohydrate: 15 gm
Protein: 6 gm
Fat: 3 gm

Sugarless Applesauce Cake

Kay Hale, Doniphan, Missouri

My mother-in-law is a diabetic, so I made this moist, spicy cake for her birthday. I also took a first place with it at our county fair!

1 cup raisins
1 cup diced dried fruit
2 cups water
2 cups all-purpose flour
1 teaspoon baking soda
1/2 teaspoon salt
1/2 teaspoon ground nutmeg
1-1/2 teaspoons ground cinnamon
Egg substitute equivalent to 2 eggs
1 cup unsweetened applesauce
2 tablespoons liquid artificial sweetener
3/4 cup vegetable oil
1 teaspoon vanilla extract
1/2 cup chopped nuts

Combine raisins, fruit and water in a saucepan; cook, uncovered, until water is evaporated and fruit is soft. Set aside to cool. Meanwhile, in a large mixing bowl, combine flour, baking soda, salt, nutmeg and cinnamon. In another bowl, combine egg substitute, applesauce, sweetener, oil and vanilla. Add nuts and fruit mixture. Stir into dry ingredients and blend thoroughly. Pour into a 10-in. fluted tube pan coated with nonstick cooking spray. Bake at 350° for 35-40 minutes or until the cake tests done. **Yield:** 32 servings.

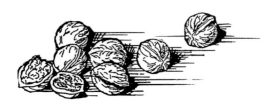

Exchanges: 1 Fat, 1/2 Starch, 1/2 Fruit
Nutritional Information

Serving Size: 1 piece
Calories: 125
Sodium: 60 mg
Cholesterol: 0

Carbohydrate: 15 gm
Protein: 2 gm
Fat: 7 gm

Prune-Pecan Cookies

Lucille Dent, Galesburg, Michigan

I like to keep these cookies on hand for unexpected company. They not only taste terrific, they're very eye-catching.

1 egg
7 dried prunes
1/2 cup sugar
1 cup all-purpose flour
1/2 teaspoon baking soda
Pinch salt
24 pecan halves

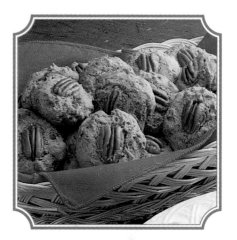

In a blender, puree egg and prunes until finely chopped. Pour into a mixing bowl. Add sugar. Combine the flour, baking soda and salt; add to prune mixture and mix well. Drop by rounded teaspoonfuls onto baking sheets coated with nonstick cooking spray. Top each cookie with a pecan half. Bake at 350° for 13-15 minutes or until golden brown. Remove to wire racks to cool. **Yield:** 2 dozen.

Exchanges: 1/2 Starch, 1/2 Fruit
Nutritional Information

Serving Size: 1 cookie
Calories: 58
Sodium: 12 mg
Cholesterol: 9 gm

Carbohydrate: 10 gm
Protein: 1 gm
Fat: 2 gm

Low-Fat Vanilla Pudding

Laura Letobar, Livonia, Michigan

I'm a radiation therapist, and I found many of my patients needed a low-fat diet. Before I knew it, I was also providing low-fat recipes to family and friends. Everyone says this dessert appears on their menus often.

1 cup skim milk
1 cup fat-free plain yogurt
1 cup fat-free sugar-free vanilla
   yogurt
1 package (1 ounce) sugar-free
   instant vanilla pudding mix
1/2 teaspoon vanilla extract
Maraschino cherries, optional
Mint leaves, optional

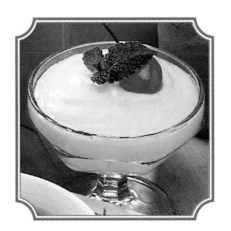

In a mixing bowl, combine milk, yogurt, pudding mix and vanilla. Beat on high speed for 2 minutes. Spoon into serving dishes. Chill. If desired, garnish with cherries and mint. **Yield:** 6 servings.

Exchanges: 1/2 Skim Milk, 1/2 Starch
Nutritional Information

Serving Size: 1/2 cup
Calories: 88
Sodium: 261 mg
Cholesterol: 3 mg

Carbohydrate: 15 gm
Protein: 5 gm
Fat: 1 gm
(Calculated without garnish)

Sugar-Free Star-Spangled Dessert

Margaret Peterson, Rothschild, Wisconsin

This dessert takes some time to prepare because each layer must set before the next is added. But I think you'll agree the festive result is worth the wait!

BOTTOM LAYER:
- 1 pint fresh *or* frozen blueberries
- 2 cups water
- 1 package (.6 ounce) sugar-free blueberry-flavored gelatin
- 1 cup cold water

MIDDLE LAYER:
- 1 envelope unflavored gelatin
- 1/2 cup cold water
- 1 cup skim milk
- 1 package (8 ounces) light cream cheese, softened
- 12 packets artificial sweetener (equivalent to 1/2 cup sugar)
- 1 teaspoon vanilla extract

TOP LAYER:
- 1 package (.6 ounce) sugar-free raspberry-flavored gelatin
- 2 cups boiling water
- 2 cups cold water

In a saucepan, simmer blueberries and water over medium heat until berries are soft. Remove from heat; stir in blueberry gelatin until dissolved. Add cold water and mix well. Pour into a 13-in. x 9-in. x 2-in. pan. Chill until set, about 40 minutes. In a small bowl, sprinkle the unflavored gelatin over cold water; let stand for 1 minute. Heat milk but do not boil; add to softened gelatin and stir to dissolve. In a mixing bowl, beat cream cheese, sweetener and vanilla until smooth. Gradually beat in milk mixture. Spoon over bottom layer. Chill until set, about 30 minutes. Dissolve raspberry gelatin in boiling water; stir in cold water. Spoon over the middle layer. Chill until set, at least 2 hours. **Yield:** 16 servings.

Exchanges: 1/2 Fruit, 1/2 Fat

Nutritional Information

Serving Size: 1 piece	Carbohydrate: 5 gm
Calories: 57	Protein: 2 gm
Sodium: 117 mg	Fat: 3 gm
Cholesterol: 8 mg	

Sugar-Free Chocolate Fudge

Kaye Hartley, Jacksonville, Florida

I am borderline diabetic so I have to watch my desserts.
This fudge appeases my sweet tooth! I also like to make this for
friends and family as a special gift from my kitchen during the holidays.

2 packages (8 ounces *each*) cream cheese, softened
2 squares (1 ounce *each*) unsweetened chocolate, melted and cooled
24 packets artificial sweetener (equivalent to 1 cup sugar)
1 teaspoon vanilla extract
1/2 cup chopped pecans

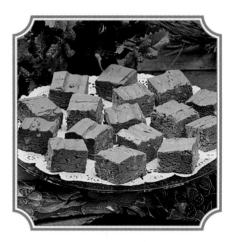

In a small mixing bowl, beat the cream cheese, chocolate, sweetener and vanilla until smooth. Stir in pecans. Pour into an 8-in. square baking pan lined with foil. Cover and refrigerate overnight. Cut into 16 squares. Serve chilled. **Yield:** 16 servings.

Exchanges: 3 Fat
Nutritional Information

Serving Size: 1 square
Calories: 147
Sodium: 84 mg
Cholesterol: 31 mg

Carbohydrate: 5 gm
Protein: 3 gm
Fat: 14 gm

Lemon Rice Pudding

Barbara Parker, Newport, New Hampshire

The addition of grated lemon peel makes this a nice change of pace from traditional rice puddings. Everyone will savor this refreshingly creamy dessert.

1-1/2 cups water
1/2 cup uncooked long grain rice
1/3 cup raisins
1/4 teaspoon ground nutmeg
1 package (1 ounce) instant sugar-free vanilla pudding mix
2 teaspoons grated lemon peel

In a saucepan, combine water, rice, raisins and nutmeg. Cover and simmer 15-20 minutes or until all liquid is absorbed. Cool. Prepare pudding mix according to package directions. Stir in rice mixture and lemon peel. Serve immediately or refrigerate. **Yield:** 7 servings.

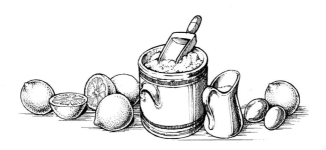

Exchanges: 1 Starch
Nutritional Information

Serving Size: 1/2 cup
Calories: 93
Sodium: 184 mg
Cholesterol: 0

Carbohydrate: 21 gm
Protein: 2 gm
Fat: 1 gm

Raisin Oatmeal Mini-Scones

Andrea Pflughaupt, Seward, Nebraska

Through the years, I've tried many sugarless dessert recipes. But these scones are by far the best. With lots of raisins and oatmeal, they make very satisfying treats.

2/3 cup margarine, melted
1-1/2 cups quick-cooking oats
Egg substitute equivalent to 2 eggs
1 teaspoon vanilla extract
Artificial sweetener equivalent to 1 cup sugar
1-1/2 cups all-purpose flour
1 teaspoon baking powder
1/2 teaspoon salt
1/2 cup skim milk
1/2 cup raisins

In a large bowl, combine margarine and oats. Stir in egg substitute, vanilla and sweetener. Combine flour, baking powder and salt; add to oat mixture alternately with milk. Stir in raisins. Drop by rounded tablespoonfuls onto baking sheets coated with nonstick cooking spray. Bake at 400° for 12-15 minutes or until browned. **Yield:** 3 dozen. **Editor's Note:** Use an artificial sweetener recommended for baking, such as Sweet 'N Low or Sweet One.

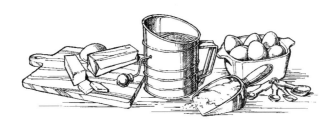

Exchanges: 1 Fat, 1/2 Starch
Nutritional Information

Serving Size: 1 scone
Calories: 77
Sodium: 83 mg
Cholesterol: trace

Carbohydrate: 9 gm
Protein: 2 gm
Fat: 4 gm

Lemon Cheesecake

Mary Merchant, Barre, Vermont

(ALSO PICTURED ON FRONT COVER)

If you're looking for a cool, creamy dessert that even a diabetic can indulge in, try this cheesecake. You'll be surprised at how wonderful it tastes. And your guests will appreciate the fact it's low in cholesterol.

1 cup graham cracker crumbs
2 tablespoons light margarine, melted
3 packages (8 ounces *each*) low-fat cream cheese, softened
2 tablespoons all-purpose flour
1/4 cup sugar
3 tablespoons fresh lemon juice
3/4 cup egg substitute
1 carton (8 ounces) sugar-free fat-free lemon yogurt
Assorted fresh berries, optional

Combine cracker crumbs and margarine; press into bottom of an ungreased 9-in. springform pan. Set aside. Beat cream cheese, flour and sugar until light and fluffy. Gradually add lemon juice and egg substitute. Beat well. Fold in yogurt. Pour into crust. Cover loosely with foil. Bake at 350° for 60-70 minutes or until center is almost set. Cool to room temperature. Refrigerate. Garnish with berries if desired. **Yield:** 16 servings.

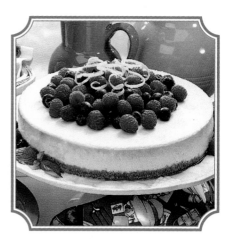

Exchanges: 1-1/2 Fat, 1 Starch, 1/2 Meat

Nutritional Information

Serving Size: 1 slice
Calories: 178
Sodium: 330 mg
Cholesterol: 25 mg

Carbohydrate: 16 gm
Protein: 7 gm
Fat: 10 gm
(Calculated without berries)

Sugar-Free Apple Pie

Teresa Garlick, Glendale, Arizona

Here's a delicious sugar-free version of a dessert that diabetics usually are forced to pass up. I guarantee your family will fall for this delicious treat.

1/3 cup frozen apple juice
   concentrate
4 packets artificial sweetener
   (equal to 8 teaspoons sugar)
2 teaspoons cornstarch
1 teaspoon ground cinnamon
Pastry for double-crust pie (9 inches)
8 cups thinly sliced peeled baking
   apples
1 tablespoon margarine

Combine the first four ingredients. Line pie plate with bottom crust; add apples. Pour juice mixture over apples; dot with margarine. Roll out remaining pastry to fit top of pie; cut slits or an apple shape in top. Place over filling; seal and flute the edges. Bake at 375° for 35 minutes. Increase temperature to 400°; bake 15-20 minutes or until apples are tender. **Yield:** 8 servings.
Editor's Note: Use an artificial sweetener recommended for baking, such as Sweet 'N Low or Sweet One.

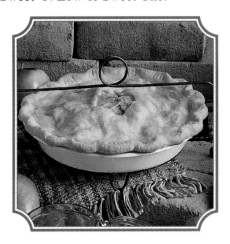

Exchanges: 3 Fat, 2 Fruit, 1 Starch

Nutritional Information

Serving Size: 1 slice
Calories: 337
Sodium: 233 mg
Cholesterol: 0

Carbohydrate: 45 gm
Protein: 2 gm
Fat: 17 gm

Condiments

*It's easy to liven up your favorite foods
with this superb selection of
salad dressings, jams, relishes…and more!*

Fresh Salsa

Myra Innes, Auburn, Kansas

This recipe uses a lot of fresh tomatoes and keeps well for several days in the refrigerator. Around our house, we like salsa as a topping for our favorite Mexican dishes and as a snack.

4 cups chopped peeled fresh
  tomatoes
1/4 cup finely chopped onion
1 to 4 jalapeno peppers,
  seeded and finely chopped
1 tablespoon olive *or*
  vegetable oil

1 tablespoon vinegar
1 teaspoon ground cumin
1 garlic clove, minced

In a bowl, combine all ingredients; mix well. Let stand for about 1 hour. Serve at room temperature. Store in a covered container in the refrigerator. **Yield:** 3-1/2 cups.

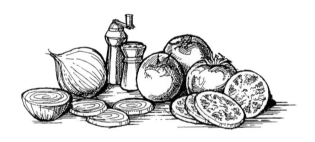

Exchanges: 1 Vegetable
Nutritional Information

Serving Size: 1/4 cup
Calories: 22
Sodium: 2 mg
Cholesterol: 0

Carbohydrate: 3 gm
Protein: 1 gm
Fat: 1 gm

Berry Good Topping

Martha Balser, Cincinnati, Ohio

The natural sweetness of fresh berries comes through in this tempting topping. I like to pour it over pancakes or ice cream. I think you'll agree it really is "berry" good!

1 pint fresh raspberries, *divided*
1/4 cup unsweetened apple juice
2 tablespoons unsweetened apple juice concentrate
2 teaspoons cornstarch
1/4 teaspoon vanilla extract

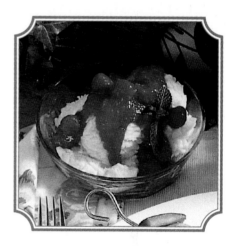

In a blender, puree 1 cup of the berries with apple juice. In a small saucepan, combine apple juice concentrate and cornstarch; stir until smooth. Add pureed berries. Cook over low heat, stirring constantly, until thickened. Cool. Add vanilla and remaining raspberries. Serve over yogurt, ice cream or pancakes. **Yield:** 8 servings (1-1/2 cups).

Exchanges: 1/2 Fruit

Nutritional Information

Serving Size: 3 tablespoons
Calories: 35
Sodium: 1 mg
Cholesterol: 0

Carbohydrate: 8 gm
Protein: 1 gm
Fat: trace

Creamy Onion Dill Dressing

Jennie Wilburn, Long Creek, Oregon

I like this dressing because it's creamy and has a great, fresh taste. We prefer it to any bottled low-fat salad dressing. You may also want to try serving this as a vegetable dip.

1 cup plain low-fat yogurt
2 tablespoons light mayonnaise
1-1/4 teaspoons snipped fresh dill
1/2 teaspoon dried parsley flakes
1/4 teaspoon garlic powder
1/8 teaspoon pepper
1/2 teaspoon low-sodium beef
  bouillon granules
1 teaspoon hot water
1 teaspoon dried minced onion

In a small bowl, mix yogurt and mayonnaise. Add dill, parsley, garlic powder and pepper. In another bowl, dissolve bouillon in water. Add onion; add to yogurt mixture and mix well. Refrigerate several hours before serving. **Yield:** 1 cup.

EASY EQUIVALENT. Do you prefer to use fresh herbs in recipes? Or does a recipe call for fresh herbs and you only have dried? No problem! The ratio for fresh herbs to dried herbs is 3 to 1. So it's easy to make substitutions in all of your favorite dishes.

Exchanges: 1/2 Vegetable, 1/2 Fat

Nutritional Information

Serving Size: 2 tablespoons
Calories: 31
Sodium: 45 mg
Cholesterol: 3 mg

Carbohydrate: 3 gm
Protein: 2 gm
Fat: 1 gm

Blueberry Jam

Fran Boise, Marion, New York

At the height of blueberry season, you'll find me making many jars of this savory jam for friends and family. Not only is it sugar-free, this jam is cholesterol-free besides. So, it's perfect for everyone!

1/2 of a 6-ounce can frozen apple
  juice concentrate, thawed
1 envelope unflavored gelatin
5 cups fresh *or* frozen
  blueberries
1 tablespoon lemon juice
1/4 teaspoon ground nutmeg
1/8 teaspoon ground cinnamon

Pour the apple juice concentrate into a saucepan; sprinkle with gelatin and allow to soften for several minutes. Meanwhile, in a blender or food processor, finely chop blueberries, 1 cup at a time. Add lemon juice, spices and 2 cups of chopped berries to gelatin; heat over medium-low until gelatin is dissolved. Remove from the heat; stir in remaining berries and mix well. Pour into jars or plastic containers; store in the refrigerator up to 3 weeks. **Yield:** 4 cups.

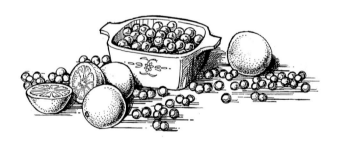

Exchanges: 1 Free Food

Nutritional Information

Serving Size: 1 tablespoon
Calories: 12
Sodium: 1 mg
Cholesterol: 0

Carbohydrate: 3 gm
Protein: trace
Fat: trace

Sugar-Free Pear Butter

Bonnie Haugen, Semmes, Alabama

*I love the flavor of pears, so I was thrilled to come across this recipe.
My family prefers this butter to traditional apple butter.*

4 quarts water
1/2 cup lemon juice, *divided*
4 pounds firm ripe pears (about
   10 large)
2/3 cup white grape juice
2 teaspoons ground cinnamon
1 teaspoon ground cloves
1/4 teaspoon ground allspice
8 to 12 packets artificial sweetener

In a kettle, combine water and 1/4 cup lemon juice. Peel, core and quarter the pears, placing them in lemon juice mixture to retard browning until all have been peeled. Drain liquid in kettle. Add grape juice and remaining lemon juice; bring to a boil. Reduce heat to medium; cook until pears are soft, about 20 minutes, stirring occasionally. Cool. Press through a sieve or food mill, or process in a blender or food processor until smooth. Return puree to kettle. Add spices; cook and stir until very thick, 20-35 minutes. Remove from heat; stir in sweetener. Adjust sweetener to taste. Pour into jars or plastic containers. Refrigerate up to 3 weeks. (For longer storage time, pour hot into hot jars, leaving 1/4-in. headspace. Process in a boiling-water bath for 10 minutes. Use within 3 weeks of opening.) **Yield:** 4 cups.

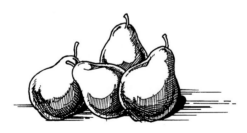

Exchanges: 1/2 Fruit

Nutritional Information

Serving Size: 1 tablespoon
Calories: 26
Sodium: 1 mg
Cholesterol: 0

Carbohydrate: 7 gm
Protein: trace
Fat: trace

Fat-Free Tartar Sauce

Laura Letobar, Livonia, Michigan

I usually keep a batch of this tartar sauce on hand to serve with all types of seafood or fish (like my Heavenly Crab Cakes on page 208). You'll be delighted with its excellent flavor!

1/2 cup fat-free plain yogurt
1/4 cup fat-free mayonnaise
  1 tablespoon sweet pickle relish, drained
  2 teaspoons dried minced onion
  1 teaspoon Dijon mustard

  1 teaspoon dried parsley flakes
  2 drops hot pepper sauce

In a small bowl, combine all ingredients. Cover and refrigerate for several hours. **Yield:** 1 cup.

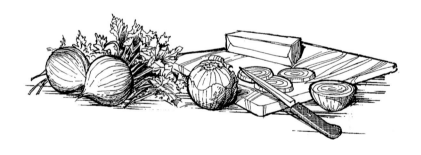

Exchanges: 1 Free Food

Nutritional Information

Serving Size: 1 tablespoon
Calories: 9
Sodium: 43 mg
Cholesterol: trace

Carbohydrate: 2 gm
Protein: trace
Fat: trace

Northwest Cherry Salsa

Margaret Slocum, Ridgefield, Washington

Among the 50 fruit trees on our place are five cherry trees—and I like to use every bit of fruit that doesn't get eaten right off of them. This recipe is one of my favorite uses for cherries.

1 cup fresh *or* frozen pitted dark
    sweet cherries, chopped
2 tablespoons chopped fresh basil
1 tablespoon finely chopped green
    pepper
1 teaspoon lemon juice
1/4 teaspoon Worcestershire sauce
1/4 teaspoon grated lemon peel
1/8 teaspoon salt
Dash hot pepper sauce

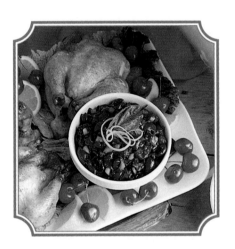

Combine all ingredients; refrigerate at least 1 hour. Serve as a condiment with chicken, turkey or pork. **Yield:** 3/4 cup.

Exchanges: 1/2 Fruit

Nutritional Information

Serving Size: 2 tablespoons
Calories: 22
Sodium: 59 mg
Cholesterol: 0

Carbohydrate: 5 gm
Protein: 1 gm
Fat: 1/2 gm

Pear Cranberry Relish

Ann Rayas, Greenville, South Carolina

Some relishes tend to be loaded with sugar, but I can enjoy this pear and cranberry version without any guilt. We like to eat it with a variety of foods.

3 cups fresh *or* frozen cranberries
1/2 cup water
5 large pears (about 2 pounds),
   peeled and cubed
1 cup orange juice
2 teaspoons grated orange peel
2 packets artificial sweetener
   (equivalent to 4 teaspoons sugar)

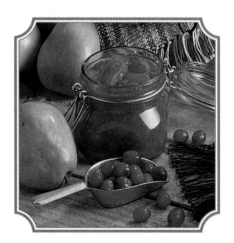

In a large saucepan, simmer cranberries in water for 10-15 minutes or until tender. Add pears, orange juice and peel; simmer 15 minutes or until tender. Cool 15 minutes. Sprinkle with sweetener; stir well. Chill for 2 hours. **Yield:** 10 servings.

Exchanges: 1 Fruit
Nutritional Information

Serving Size: 1/3 cup
Calories: 75
Sodium: 1 mg
Cholesterol: 0 mg

Carbohydrate: 19 gm
Protein: 1 gm
Fat: trace

Sugar-Free Strawberry Jam

Rita Christ, Wauwatosa, Wisconsin

My husband's been a diabetic for over 20 years. He was tired of eating the flavorless jams for diabetics in the grocery store, so I came up with this recipe. With its fresh flavor, it makes a nice gift.

3/4 cup diet lemon-lime soda
1 package (.3 ounce) sugar-free
**   strawberry-flavored gelatin**
1 cup mashed fresh *or*
**   unsweetened frozen strawberries**
1-1/2 teaspoons lemon juice

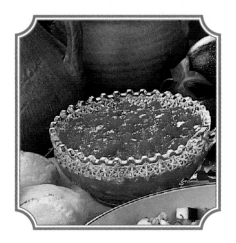

In a saucepan, bring soda to a boil. Remove from the heat; stir in gelatin until dissolved. Stir in strawberries and lemon juice. Pour into jars or plastic containers; cover and refrigerate up to 3 weeks. Do not freeze. **Yield:** 1-3/4 cups.

Exchanges: 1 Free Food
Nutritional Information

Serving Size: 1 tablespoon
Calories: 4
Sodium: 9 mg
Cholesterol: 0

Carbohydrate: 1 gm
Protein: trace
Fat: trace

Low-Fat Italian Dressing

Shonna Lee Leonard, Sackville, Nova Scotia

*Most Italian dressings are laden with oil and fat. So,
when I found this recipe years ago, I knew I had to try it.
Now I make it often for my family. They love it!*

5 tablespoons frozen apple juice
  concentrate, thawed
1/4 cup cider vinegar
1/4 cup lemon juice
1 garlic clove, minced
1/2 teaspoon *each* onion powder,
  paprika, dried mustard and
  oregano

1/4 teaspoon dried basil
1/8 teaspoon dried thyme
1/8 teaspoon dried rosemary,
  crushed

In a jar with a tight-fitting lid, mix all ingredients. Chill several hours or overnight.
Shake well before serving. **Yield:** 3/4 cup.

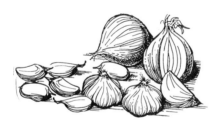

Exchanges: 1/2 Fruit
Nutritional Information
Serving Size: 2 tablespoons
Calories: 30
Sodium: 6 mg
Cholesterol: 0

Carbohydrate: 8 gm
Protein: trace
Fat: trace

Low-Fat Ranch Dressing

Cindy Bertrand, Floydada, Texas

*This creamy, rich-tasting dressing is a very deceiving low-fat alternative!
And people are surprised to see the short list of ingredients called for
in this recipe. Everyone thinks a delicious
dressing like this would take hours to prepare.*

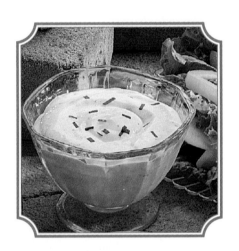

**1 package (2 ounces) low-fat
  ranch salad dressing mix**
1-1/2 cups skim milk
1/4 cup fat-free sour cream
1/4 cup fat-free mayonnaise

In a small bowl, combine all ingredients
until smooth. Cover and chill. Serve over
salad greens. Keep refrigerated. **Yield:** 2
cups.

Exchanges: 1 Free Food

Nutritional Information

Serving Size: 2 tablespoons
Calories: 26
Sodium: 263 mg
Cholesterol: 1 mg

Carbohydrate: 4 gm
Protein: 1 gm
Fat: trace

Cranberry Apple Relish

Carla Hodenfield, Mandan, North Dakota

Give this tart, rose-colored relish a try. It really enhances the flavor of turkey and chicken. It's a special dish even for those who can have sugar.

**2 cups ground fresh *or* frozen
   cranberries**
1/2 cup diced peeled apple
1/4 cup raisins
**2 tablespoons liquid artificial
   sweetener**
1/2 teaspoon lemon juice

In a bowl, combine all ingredients. Refrigerate for at least 2 hours. **Yield:** 10 servings.

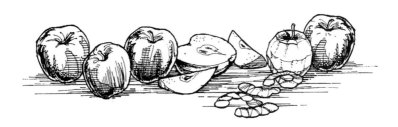

Exchanges: 1/2 Fruit
Nutritional Information

Serving Size: 1/4 cup
Calories: 24
Sodium: 1 mg
Cholesterol: 0

Carbohydrate: 6 gm
Protein: trace
Fat: trace

Index